MW00930246

# SPANISH FLU 1918

*Data and Reflections On The Consequences Of Great Influenza Pandemic,*

*What History Teaches, How Not To Repeat The Same Mistakes*

1

## © Copyright 2020 by Oscar Harwey
## All rights reserved.

This document is geared towards providing exact and reliable information concerning the topic and issue covered. The publication is sold with the idea that the publisher is not required to render accounting, officially permitted or otherwise qualified services. If advice is necessary, legal or professional, practiced individuals in the profession should be ordered.

- From a Declaration of Principles which was accepted and approved equally by a Committee of the American Bar Association and a Committee of Publishers and Associations.

In no way is it legal to reproduce, duplicate, or transmit any part of this document in either electronic means or printed format. Recording of this publication is strictly prohibited, and any storage of this document is not allowed unless with written permission from the publisher. All rights reserved.

The information provided herein is stated to be truthful and consistent, in that any liability, in terms of inattention or otherwise, by any usage or abuse of any policies, processes, or directions contained within is the sole and utter responsibility of the recipient reader. Under no circumstances will any legal responsibility or blame be held against the publisher for any reparation, damages, or monetary loss due to the information herein, either directly or indirectly.

Respective authors own all copyrights not held by the publisher.

The information herein is offered for informational purposes solely and is universal as so. The presentation of the information is without a contract or any type of guarantee assurance.

The trademarks that are used are without any consent, and the publication of the trademark is without permission or backing by the trademark owner. All trademarks and brands within this book are for clarifying purposes only and are owned by the owners themselves, and not affiliated with this document

# Table of Contents

7

# INTRODUCTION

The Spanish Influenza pandemic is

the most lethal pandemics of the Modern Age. The number of deaths that it produced throughout the world was estimated at 21.5 million (Jordan, 1927) and 39.3 million (Patterson and Pyle, 1991). Other researchers have proposed even higher figures, which seem to be somewhat excessive. Nevertheless, the appearance and development of the Spanish Influenza continue to present several unanswered questions, which should be addressed in the light of the new influenza pandemics which have appeared at the beginning of the present XXI century, including avian influenza and the swine influenza [A/swine (H1N1)], which are considered by some, such as Taubenberger et al. (2005, 2006) or Smith et al. (2009), to be directly related to the Spanish Influenza.

The first pandemic wave, which was benign and caused few deaths, begin in the spring of 1918. After a period of calm at the beginning of the summer of 1918, the virus mutated, becoming extremely virulent, and simultaneously caused millions of deaths throughout the world during October and November. A milder third wave occurred early months of 1919, while the fourth and final wave spread during the first months of 1920. The majority of those who died were young, healthy adults between the ages of 15 and 44. Mortality rates varied between countries and continents, but mortality in Europe has been estimated to be 1.1% (Ansart et al., 2009) and 1.2% (Erkoreka, 2006).

Our principal concern in this book is to examine the historical aspect of the pandemic, its consequences (economic and social), the government and people's reaction, possible vaccines against the flu, historical lessons learned, etc.

# CHAPTER ONE

# THE EPIC STORY OF THE SPANISH FLU

# 1918

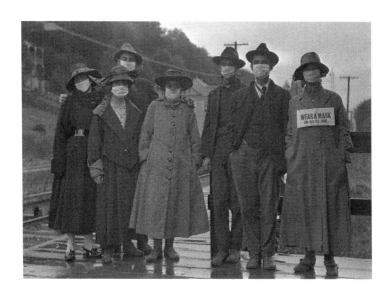

## What Is the Flu?

Influenza, or flu, is a virus that attacks the respiratory system.

The flu virus is extremely contagious: respiratory droplets are produced and spread into the air as an infected person coughs, sneezes or talks, and may then be inhaled by anyone nearby.

In fact, anyone who touches something with the virus on it and then touches his or her mouth, eyes, or nose can get contaminated. In 1918, an influenza outbreak known as Spanish flu sparked a worldwide pandemic, escalated quickly and indiscriminately murdering men. Young, elderly, disabled, and mostly safe individuals were all infected, and at least 10 percent of patients were killed.

Estimates vary on the total amount of deaths caused by the epidemic. Still, one-third of the world's population is believed to have been contaminated, and at least 50 million people killed, rendering it the worst pandemic in recent history. While it earned the label "Spanish flu" at that moment, it's doubtful that the epidemic originated from Spain.

**What caused Spanish flu?**

Influenza is triggered by many closely associated viruses, but one form (type A) is tied to deadly epidemics. The pandemic of 1918-19 originated from a disease A virus known as H1N1. Before being recognized as the Spanish flu, in the final year of World War I, the first cases reported occurred in the United States.

By March 1918, the United States was 11 months at war with Germany and the Imperial Powers. By this time, the meager, pre-war army of America, had developed into a massive fighting power that would finally send more than two million people to Europe.

As the entire nation prepared for war, American forts experienced major expansion. It was Fort Riley, Kansas, where a modern preparation center, Camp Funston, was designed to accommodate some of the 50,000 people who were to be inducted into the Army. It was there a feverish soldier returned to the infirmary early in March. Within a few hours, more than a hundred troops had come down with a similar condition, and over the ensuing weeks, more fall sick. More infected American forces landed in Europe in March. Then the pandemic's First Surge begins.

In the final months of World War I, the epidemic occurred in 1918, and historians still believe that the war might have been partially responsible for transmitting the infection. Soldiers working in hot, filthy, and unhealthy environments on the Western Front have become sick. It was a possible product of undernourished damaged digestive systems. Illnesses were contagious and dispersed throughout the ranks, known as "la grippe." Most troops would start getting stronger after only three days of becoming ill, although not everyone would make it.

As soldiers started to return home on leave during the summer of 1918, they took with them the undetected infection that had made them sick. The epidemic traveled through towns, communities, and villages throughout the homelands of the soldiers. Most of those affected, including troops and people, were not able to heal. The virus was most serious on young adults aged 20 to 30 who had previously healthy.

A new hypothesis about the virus' roots suggested it first appeared in China in 2014, National Geographic published. Previously undiscovered documents connected flu to the 1917 and 1918 transportation of Chinese labor corps in Canada. According to Mark Humphries 'book "The Last Plague" (University of Toronto Press, 2013), the laborers were mainly field employees from isolated rural China. They spent six days in enclosed train containers as they were shipped around the country before heading on to France. There they had to dig pits, unload trains, lay paths, construct roads and rebuild tanks that were destroyed. In total, the Western Sector has recruited more than 90,000 personnel.

Humphries states that in 1918, about 3,000 in one estimation of 25,000 Chinese workers began their Canadian trip in medical quarantine. Throughout the moment, their sickness was blamed on "Asian laziness" because of racist prejudices, and Canadian physicians could not treat the complaints of the staff seriously. At the time the workforce landed in northern France in early 1918, many had been ill, and soon hundreds were dying.

## Why was it called Spanish flu?

Spain was one of the first countries in which the disease was reported, but scholars agree that this was a result of repression during the conflict. Throughout the conflict, Spain became a democratic country and did not impose rigid control

in the newspapers, which would, therefore, be able to print early reports of the outbreak. As a consequence, citizens mistakenly thought the illness was Spanish-specific, and the term "Spanish flu" remained.

According to Henry Davies 'book "The Spanish Flu," (Henry Holt & Co., 2000), also in late Spring 1918, a Spanish news service sent word to Reuters' London office telling the news agency that "a peculiar type of infectious fever has arisen in Madrid. The outbreak is of a mild sort, no deaths have been recorded." More than 100,000 people had been sick with the flu within two weeks of the study.

The illness affected Spain's King Alfonso XIII as well as leading politicians. Infected between 30% and 40% of citizens who served or resided in enclosed environments, such as schools, hospitals, and government offices. There was a need to cut operation on the Madrid train network, and the telegraph operation was interrupted in all situations as there was no sufficient staff willing to operate. Health equipment and facilities are incapable of satisfying demand.

In Britain, the term "Spanish influenza" soon took control. According to Niall Johnson's book "Britain and the Influenza Pandemic of 1918-19" (Routledge, 2006), the British press blamed the Spanish weather for the flu outbreak in Spain: "... the hot, windy Spanish spring is an unpredictable and dangerous season," read one report in The Times. It was reported that the high winds in Spain were blowing microbe-laden spores, which suggests the rainy environment in Britain might avoid the flu from blowing there.

## What were the symptoms of the flu?

Early symptoms of the illness involved sore head and fatigue, accompanied by dry, hacking cough; lack of appetite; stomach problems, and finally, heavy sweating on the second day. First, the disease may impact the pulmonary organs and can cause pneumonia. Humphries states that the major causes of mortality were mostly pneumonia or other respiratory problems induced by the flu. This is why precise figures affected by the flu became impossible to ascertain, as the reported cause of death was sometimes anything other than the flu.

Over the summer of 1918, the epidemic spread quickly to many continental European countries such as Vienna, Budapest, and Hungary, and also impacted areas in Germany and France. Several children were registered sick and absent from school in Berlin schools, and productivity was decreased by absences in armament factories.

The Spanish flu outbreak had entered Britain by June 25, 1918. According to "The Spanish Influenza Pandemic of 1918-1919: Modern Perspectives," the outbreak struck the

London clothing industry hard in July, with one plant seeing 80 out of 400 staff heading home sick in one evening alone (Routledge 2003). In London, estimates of missing government employees owing to flu vary from 25 to 50 percent of the population.

The outbreak has soon developed into a pandemic, finding its way around the world. Six Canadian warships were drowned on the St. Lawrence River in August 1918. Cases were registered among the Swedish Army in the same month, then among the civilian population of the world and even among the laboring community of South Africa. The flu had entered the U.S. via Boston harbor by September.

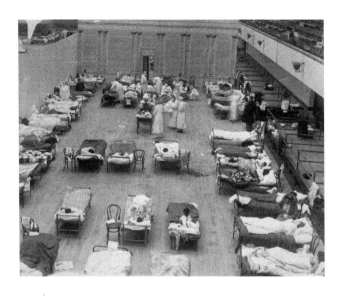

## Deadly Virus

The Spanish flu strain destroyed its victims with unparalleled swiftness. There were lots of people turning up ill and dead on their way to work in United States reports. The signs were gruesome: patients would run a fever and be out of air. Oxygen depletion indicated that their faces looked tinged with grey. Blood flooded the bloodstream with hemorrhages, inducing severe diarrhea and nosebleeds, with patients swimming in their fluids. Like too many influenza viruses before it, Spanish flu affected not just the very young and the very elderly but also stable people aged between 20 and 40.

The key influence in the propagation of the virus was, of course, still in its final stages, the world crisis. The precise sources of the infection are still debated by epidemiologists. However, there is some evidence that it was the result of a genetic error that could have originated in China. But what is evident is that due to the vast and accelerated deployment of troops around the planet, the current challenge was going worldwide.

The war excitement has often helped to mask the latest virus's exceptionally high mortality levels. The disease was not fully known at the initial point, and fatalities had also been due to pneumonia. Strict wartime censorship means that outbreaks could not be published in the European and North American press. The press could write openly about what was occurring

and in neutral Spain, and it was from this public attention that the disease received its title.

## What advice were people given?

Physicians were at a loss as to what to recommend to their patients; several doctors advised people to avoid crowded places or just other people. Some remedies suggested include eating cinnamon, consuming wine, or even consuming meat from Oxo (beef broth). Doctors have even advised citizens to keep their ears and eyes closed voluntarily. At one point, aspirin usage was blamed for triggering the pandemic, although it may have potentially benefited those affected.

A public note published in the British papers on June 28, 1918, warning citizens of the effects of flu; however, it turned out that this was, in reality, advertising for Formamints, a supplement manufactured and marketed by a vitamin firm. Just when people were suffering, there was money to be gained from bogus "cures" ads. The commercial claimed that the mints were the "only way of stopping contagious diseases" and that everybody, including babies, would suck four to five of such tablets a day before they feel stronger.

Specific guidance was given to Americans about how to stop being infected. They were told not to shake hands with anyone, remain indoors, avoid touching books from libraries, and wear masks. According to a study released in the journal Public Health Studies, schools and theatres reopened, and the New York City Department of Health specifically applied an update to the Sanitary Code that made vomiting into the streets unlawful.

In some areas, World War I ended due to the shortage of physicians, and many of the patients are remaining sick. Schools and other structures were makeshift clinics, and in some instances, medical students had to assume the place of physicians.

## How many people died?

At the beginning of 1919, the mortality rate from Spanish flu declined. Countries were left ravaged in the aftermath of the epidemic because medical practitioners did not escape the disease spread. The pandemic mirrored what occurred 500 years ago when the Black Death wreaked global havoc.

Nancy Bristow's book "American Pandemic: The Forgotten Dimensions of the 1918 Influenza Outbreak" (Oxford University Press, 2016) states that as many as 500 million individuals worldwide have been infected by the infection that constituted one-third of the world's population at the time while the actual number is believed to be much larger, as many as 50 million people have suffered from the infection.

Bristow reports that as many as 25 percent of the U.S. populace and members of the U.S. navy become contaminated with the virus, this figure reached up to 40%, likely owing to sea service conditions. At the end of October 1918, the flu had claimed the lives of 200,000 Americans, and Bristow says the pandemic had destroyed over 675,000 Americans overall. The effect on the population was so severe that life expectancy was decreased by 12 years in 1918.

Bodies piled up to the extent that cemeteries were crowded, and families were compelled to dig graves for their ancestors. The losses culminated in a lack of farm workers, impacting the late summer harvest. In Germany, other facilities, such as waste disposal, are being placed under strain from a shortage of workforce and funding.

The pandemic spread to Asia, Latin America, Africa, and the South Pacific. The mortality rate in India exceeded 50 deaths per 1,000 population, and this was a staggering and disturbing amount.

## The second wave

The overcrowded First World War trenches and encampments were the prime habitats for this epidemic. But the virus went with them as troops marched. Within a few weeks, the storm that had first erupted in Kansas weakened, but that was just a brief relief. Through September 1918, the epidemic was poised to hit the worst phase.

It has been estimated that the 13 weeks between September and December 1918 were the most intense time, claiming the most lives. In October alone, at least 195,000 Americans died. In contrast, overall American military losses come in at just over 116,000 for the entirety of World War I. Again, and it was the noisy military encampments that the second wave acquired a grip at first, 6,674 cases had been recorded at Camp Devens, a Massachusetts military base, in September.

The medical services started to get exhausted as the epidemic hit its zenith. Morticians and gravediggers suffered, and it became difficult to execute private funerals. Most of those who perished ended up in mass graves. The end of 1918 saw a lull in the outbreak of the epidemic, with the advent of the third and final period in January 1919. At that time, the epidemic had become a much-weakened power. The prior year's autumn and winter ferocity were not replicated, so death levels reduced.

While the final wave was much less deadly than its counterparts, it was nevertheless able to cause significant damage. Australia, which had soon imposed quarantine controls, continued to avoid the worst of the flu by the beginning of 1919 when the epidemic eventually came and brought several thousand Australians to their homes.

Nevertheless, the overall mortality trend had been downward. There were reports of influenza deaths — possibly a new strain — as late as 1920. Still, the free treatment programs and the virus 'inevitable genetic evolution put the disease to an end by the summer of 1919. And then, its consequences were to last decades for many left bereaved or enduring problems of long-term safety.

### How does this compare to seasonal flu?

Having destroyed approximately 1 to 3 percent of the world's population, Spanish flu is the most lethal flu pandemic to date by far.

The most recent comparable flu pandemic happened in 2009-2010, following the introduction of a modern version of the

H1N1 influenza virus. Since the virus triggers it is identical to the one present in pigs (not that the virus comes from pigs), the illness was called "swine flu."

According to the Centers for Disease Prevention and Control, the swine flu triggered respiratory diseases, which killed an estimated 151,700-575,400 people worldwide in the first year. That was about 0.001 or 0.007 percent of the world's population, and this pandemic was much less impactful than the Spanish flu pandemic of 1918. About 80 percent of swine flu fatalities resulted among individuals younger than 65, which was unprecedented. Usually, 70 to 90 percent of severe influenza-related fatalities occur in individuals older than 65 years.

An influenza strain vaccine that causes swine flu is now included in the annual flu vaccines. Every year people often suffer from the flu, but the figures are significantly smaller, on average than those for swine flu or Spanish flu pandemics.

According to the International Health Organisation, global severe flu epidemics end in around 3 million to 5 million serious illness events and between 290,000 to 650,000 fatalities.

## Genetic characterization of the 1918 'Spanish' influenza virus

By the end of the First World War, in the fall of 1918, the globe was engulfed by an influenza pandemic with unparalleled virulence, with as many as 40 million dead in its midst. This virus claimed the lives of many healthy young people around the world. At that moment, the virus that was responsible for this tragedy was not known, and maybe the most deadly infectious agent of all moment was unavailable for research. The quest for the agent responsible for the pandemic began earnestly in 1918 and culminated in the discovery of the first influenza virus in swine in 1930 and humans in 1933, 12 years later. Following 70 years of research shone a lot of light on influenza virus biology, but still unresolved questions remain. The genetic characteristics of the 1918 virus can now be researched due to the remarkable foresight of the US Army Medical Museum, the dedication of pathologist Johan V. Hultin, and the developments in molecular genetic analysis of defined tissue specimens as demonstrated by the Molecular Pathology Division at the Washington, D.C. Armed Forces Institute of Pathology.

The 1918 virus study isn't just one of the historical curiosities. Since influenza viruses are constantly evolving through antigenic change and drift processes, new influenza strains continue to endanger human populations as emerging pathogenic elements. Since 1918, pandemic influenza viruses developed twice, in 1957 and 1968. There is a perceived strong chance of potential influenza pandemics. These potential pandemics may be encouraged by an awareness of the genetic make- of the most virulent influenza strain in history.

## Indirect information on the virus

Analysis of 1918 flu survivors 'antibody titers from the late 1930s and historical phylogenetic research indicates that the 1918 strain was an H1N1 subtype influenza A virus, most strongly linked to what is now known as the' modern swine 'influenza virus. The swine relation also specifically relates to the flu of 1918, during the second wave, widespread influenza outbreaks of humans and pigs were recorded all over the world.

While historical records indicate that the 1918 flu spread from humans to pigs, the interaction between these two animals in the 1918 flu has not been resolved. However, no assessment was made on the avian connection with the 1918 flu. A wild waterfowl are considered to be the main source of the influenza virus. In species resistant to humans, genetic material from avian organisms appears regularly. Since pigs may be contaminated with both avian and human pathogens, in this cycle, they have been postulated as intermediaries. Avian influenza A virus (without reassortment) joined the swine community of northern Europe of 1979, establishing a strong group of viruses. Influenza viruses with genetic material newly obtained were responsible for the outbreaks of pandemic influenza in 1957 and 1968. There was no proof until it was recently confirmed that a complete avian influenza virus could directly infect humans. The barrier was significantly breached in Hong Kong in 1997 when at least eighteen people became diagnosed with an avian H5N1 influenza virus, and six died as a result of complications.

One of the main aims of this project is the relationship of the 1918 influenza virus to swine and avian viral strains. Whether influenza viruses pass between organisms is critically critical to our knowledge of the pandemic influenza strains that arise.

## The Power of Gender during the Influenza pandemic in the United States

In the fall of 1918, Fort Des Moines 'student nurses replied to a request for action, entering the war against widespread influenza and then spreading across the midwest of the Americas. Recording her classmates 'encounters in the school yearbook, one girl, Mabel Chilson, remembered the dedication with which she and her cohorts approached the debilitating illness. 'We asked, "Are we powerless, or were we willing to fight? "We joined the ranks with willing resolve." While at work, according to Chilson, the nurses 'soon became the best team, and we had amusing good times while off of service.

The greatest comfort we enjoyed was the understanding that each girl tried her utmost and performed well as a nurse. 'Though challenged by the outbreak, Chilson and her colleagues sought affirmation as women and nurses in their work.

These nurses responded to a desperate need as they joined in the fight against the epidemic. A few months before, as the influenza outbreak first entered the United States, it had devastated a country whose store of both nurses and physicians was greatly reduced as a consequence of the war. Its powers exhausted by the demands of the war now confronted the most significant outbreak in the history of the world, healthcare professionals like Chilson. While influenza has become a frequent annual guest, this form was horrifyingly distinct from its predecessors. Striking at a speed previously unprecedented, influenza often ravaged patients within hours in the autumn of 1918, and cities subdued within days.

The epidemic had reached perhaps the most remote areas in the United States, only weeks after its introduction. This virus, which spread rapidly, was also surprisingly lethal. The outbreak had killed well over 500,000 people, increasing the average estimate of influenza. Its injuries were indeed rare. While influenza was fatal at times, it mostly hit hardest among the very young and the very elderly. However, this time influenza struck young people, many with unique virulence that is normally better prepared to withstand extreme cases of influenza. And eventually, although fatalities were attributed to several reasons, specific signs were always alarming, including, for example, severe discoloration, labored breathing, a bleeding or sputum-cough, and a blue or purple- face, the latter being the product of patients drowning in their body fluids.

In the light of this ghastly disease and its outbreak manifestation, Nurse Chilson's positive response to her encounters is remarkable, considering the degree to which identical responses were reported by other nurses. During the outbreak, Mabel Chilson's sense of frustration with nursing actions was expressed in the diaries, letters, and more widely released accounts of nurses around the Country. While acknowledging the severity of the disease and the wretched condition of its patients, nurses also offered a hopeful account of their roles in the outbreak, emphasizing the promise it provided for effective ministry.

Throughout the outbreak, doctors and nurses worked closely together, but most physician reports expressed no common sense of fulfillment. 'Influenza, you can't do much,' one professional guy admitted years back. Ignorant of the etiology of the illness, unaware of the appropriate preventive strategies and powerless to halt the spreading outbreak, physicians frequently shared a feeling of helplessness as people and modesty as leaders of a discipline.

This requires an explanation of why doctors and nurses could react so differently to their shared work during the epidemic. In 1918, healthcare in the U.S. became the domain of two separate occupations- nursing- these careers became characterized, at least in part, by the practitioners 'assumed gender identification. The medical profession has been an almost entirely male possession, with women being nursed the appropriate substitute. Then, when doctors and nurses reacted to the outbreak in 1918, they did so in the sense of a sex- medical system in which the function and obligations of health care professionals were influenced by gender. This is this gendering in healthcare roles that further describes the different responses exhibited by physicians and nurses to their interactions during the outbreak by providing doctors and nurses with widely different standards for evaluating their achievements.

Medicine hadn't always been the province of men. During the early years of the American colony, men and women shared the treatment of the sick. Nevertheless, by the late eighteenth century, a growing number of physicians started to picture themselves as members of a more prestigious occupation, focused this identification on academic preparation. It was in this sense that male medical practitioners moved to remove women from the practice. The dispute for the personal image continued throughout the nineteenth century. 'Regular' physicians, those affiliated with allopathic medicine that governs professional practice in the United States today, encountered intense pressure from several sources – from Americans who tended to focus on lay providers to practitioners to alternative types to 'irregular' medicine that involved treatments varying from nutritional counseling to hydropathy and homeopathy.

Both men and women had continued to play prominent roles in healthcare provision in this context. However, in 1918 the 'regulars' had strengthened their influence in the medical profession and developed a position of prominence in American society for themselves. Around the same moment, they have attempted to remove all but a few people from medical practice. When male physicians over the nineteenth century formed a professional image, the identification became gradually synonymous with the masculinity of the doctor. The change was accompanied by parallel nursing changes. Nursing became professionalized in the closing years of the nineteenth century. And the rise of nursing from family duty to a paying occupation did nothing to alter its status as 'the work of a woman.' Nevertheless, the rise of the nursing profession has major consequences for women's role in medicine.

These gendered notions of American healthcare were strongly developed by the time of the flu epidemic, which offered the criteria by which Americans, including carers, which laypeople alike, should measure the success of physicians and nurses.

When the epidemic struck in 1918, Americans expressed their faith quickly in the ability of modern medicine and its practitioners to protect them from serious harm. 'There would not appear to be an occasion for great concern or distress on the issue,' one newspaper editor explained in October 1918, 'because the epidemic is something that the American medical community is fully capable of coping with.' As proof of their faith in the effectiveness of conventional medicine and the abilities of its practitioners, Americans granted the medical profession considerable power to combat it.

Whereas the progression of the disease seriousness was often downplayed by public health boards and policymakers, doctors quickly understood the 'scourge' of influenza and the threat posed by its disease form. Confronted with a rare outbreak in its intensity, physicians were compelled to realize just how little they knew about influenza.

Throughout the epidemic, medical authorities ranging from the U.S. Surgeon General and some physicians writing in the American Medical Association Journal were compelled to accept that influenza 'causative cause' remained a mystery. Uncertain over the origin of the acute disease, physicians were also unable to describe the subsequent influenza-accompanying diseases, which were sometimes blamed for the deaths of patients.

With no clear understanding of the disease's etiology, doctors found an enigmatic treatment, though not for lack of effort on the part of American scientists. Many physicians focused their thoughts and efforts into creating a flu vaccine. Scientists 'quest for a remedy was likely to prove fruitless because of the lack of understanding and the origin of the disease.

By November 1918, the American Medical Association Journal editors warned Americans against putting their trust in vaccinations. The U.S. Public Health Service decided early, informing People of the possible risks involved with the vaccination, and recognizing that there was no solution available yet.

Confused both by the disease and the epidemic, doctors had already admitted that they could not affect either one. Noting the heated disagreements between doctor and student, one student recognized the inadequacy of scientific expertise mirrored these differences: it was openly accepted by all of us at sea that we are on the correct strategies of diagnosis, cure, and prevention; that we do not yet know how to deter and manage the spread of the disease, and that much of the methods used in fighting are still unknown.

Stating it clearly, as one doctor said, 'There was little you could do.' Incapable of preventing either the illness or the plague, physicians also admitted that their practitioners had nothing to give. As one doctor recalled, "There wasn't anything that a doctor might do. Before he might see him again, the guy will be gone. And still, 'The biggest task to do every day was to figure out who was dead and what kills them.' Powerless until the sickness, some doctors believed that their therapeutic attempts were futile. 'Listening to the testimonies of many health officers that their attempts to fight the disease seemed in vain, irrespective of what they did,' one doctor wrote at the end of 1918, 'I almost came to the impression that our war against the outbreak was pointless.' Many physicians also feared that their willingness to deal with the ill could do more damage than good. In this case, some doctors suggested, 'The only thing the doctor will do for the patient is to leave the patient alone.'

This feeling of powerlessness was completely surprising for others. Sure about the efficacy of germ theory, secure in its experimental methodology and proud of recent advances in the area, by the early twentieth century, several physicians had established confidence in medicine's capacity to manage any scourge. As one source immediately after the outbreak described, 'The most surprising aspect about the pandemic was the complete ambiguity around it. Technology, which has done too much to push many plagues to the point of elimination by the patient and excruciating labor, has so far been helpless before it. 'Influenza appeared to contradict the advances achieved by science and the recent claim to mastery of disease.

Confronted with the fact that this epidemic was outside their control, many physicians have shared a new sense of their profession's limits. One analyst argued that in the current crisis, 'established medical science was at fault,' while another identified 'the complete collapse of the country's public health administrations.' Although some physicians tried to preserve the efficacy of their practice during the outbreak, these reactions were uncommon.

The most popular were expressions of fear, followed by deceit and modesty, reactions which often represented a dramatic shift in the personal or professional self-image of an individual. 'It's disappointing that until the big influenza outbreak, the epidemiologist was ineffective,' one doctor commented. 'Such obstacles as we tried to put in the path of their spread have been swept away like chaff before a mighty tempest.' Frustrated by the profession's success, some practitioners preferred to condemn medicine for its ignorance. One specialist wrote an article entitled 'A General Confession by a Continent's Public Health Officials' in which Victor C. Vaughan, a prominent epidemiologist, said, 'The saddest aspect of my career was when I observed the hundreds of deaths of soldiers in the army camps and didn't know what to do. Since that moment, I never wanted to think again for the great achievements of medical science, and in this situation, humbly confess our profound ignorance.

Having once retained the heroic image of medicine, this field leader exchanged a tentative modesty for his former celebration. For others, like Vaughan, the response to the outbreak and the inability of medicine to control either the illness or the outbreak was very severe and continued to torment them even after the epidemic's disaster had ended.

Recalling memories, he felt he could never forget, Vaughan wrote in his memoirs: I see hundreds of young, stalwart people walking into hospital wards in groups of ten or more in their country's uniform. They are put on the cots when all beds are full and even more are crowded in. The faces soon spot a bluish cast; the blood-soaked sputum puts out a distressing cough. In the morning, the deceased bodies are like cordwood and are piled around the morgue. I drew this image on my memory cells. In 1918, when fatal influenza showed that human inventions were deficient in the loss of human life.

Others decided they should never overlook the epidemic's terrifying sounds or their failure to contain it. Mystified by the illness and powerless to slow down the outbreak or rescue their patients, physicians considered the outbreak often frustrating. They mostly viewed it as an experience in fear and modesty.

Acting alongside physicians, nurses often expressed the spirit of fear when they observed the damage caused by the disease, and accepted that such images would stick with them forever. As one nurse, Anna C. Jamme, remembered her first visit to a military flu hospital, "From the moment I boarded the train, I saw the horrible expression of fear in the face of everyone I saw the wards remain silent with death's stillness. It was a sight that could never be overlooked. 'While recognizing how horrific the outbreak had been, Jamme's response to what she witnessed and its effect on her view of her career is somewhat different than those shared by other physicians. Describing nurses 'rising to their duties like brave warriors' and describing her nurses 'gratitude earned from commanding officers, Jamme expressed her respect for the nurses' 'splendid service' throughout the epidemic.

Others reacted too. 'The epidemic's good memories are numerous,' wrote Eunice H. Dyke. 'The list of treasured encounters,' she concluded, 'is lengthy.' While none were as emotional as Dyke, the epidemic's nurses 'memories, at least those they documented, were not as utterly pessimistic as those of doctors. Although most reflected the sorrow and even disgust of the doctors at the pain and death they experienced, this dismay was also combined with more positive associations in their lives with this time.

That nurses have been able to recall their jobs so much more profoundly after those months reflects how deeply they perceived what they had done during the outbreak, and awareness directly related to their ideas of nursing and womanhood.

Most significantly, nurses also thought they had been able to do more good during the epidemic, offering positive care to their patients. The feeling of achievement of the nurses also represented a performance that was as easy as providing essential warmth. Describing a Red Cross nurse's job in the

Virginia mountains, one account outlined how the necessary critical treatment was, saying, 'You can understand what it meant for these men. Seeing a competent, obedient woman unexpectedly appear in their midst, and without any preliminaries to make them happy – a real angel of grace in a cap and an apron. 'Simply providing shelter for nurses was an accomplishment and one deserving of the angels.

Many sources praised much larger successes, indicating such basic actions played a major role in the recovery of patients. As suggested by Clara D. Noyes, Acting Director of the Red Cross Department of Nursing, 'The research done by the Nursing Service was breathtaking at this period. The death toll in the U.S. was massive, over 400,000. It would be difficult to say whether it might have been without a coordinated nursing service.'48 Nurses did not claim that they had healed influenza or prevented the epidemic; nevertheless, they believed that their ministries had proved valuable and rendered a significant contribution to the well-being of patients.

Nurses seemed to think their experience during the outbreak had shown both the value and the standard of nursing in the United States, and so nurses left the outbreak with an improved appreciation of their career.

The nurses' responses to the outbreak, confident of their work, have also been optimistic. 'I am so glad to know that I can help,' exclaimed one volunteer nurse. Others, too, professed their joy that they could do a nurse's job. Recalling the death of a volunteer nurse after just eight days, a study from the Red Cross highlighted the happiness that the young woman had found in her job: 'In the last moments she claimed that she had achieved more pleasure from her job over the previous eight (days) than she had in the twenty-five years of her life.' 'It was a most terrible and yet most beautiful encounter,' described one lady. Though deeply saddened, in her observations during the outbreak, this nurse saw beauty and nobility.

# CHAPTER TWO

# SOCIO-ECONOMIC CONSEQUENCES OF

# THE DEADLIEST PLAGUE

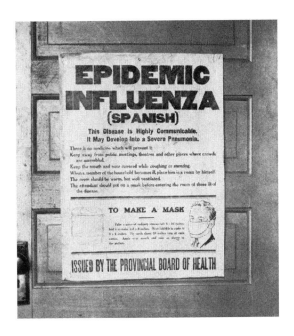

In several countries across the world, the threat of a global influenza pandemic (e.g., avian flu) in the near future is of growing interest. The World Bank estimates that a global influenza pandemic would cost $800 billion to the world economy and destroy hundreds of millions of U.S. researchers. Centers for Disease Control and Prevention report that fatalities in the U.S. will exceed 207,000, and the overall loss to the nation will be equal to $166 billion, or around 1.5 percent of GDP. The rate of long runs is projected to be significantly higher. The U.S. Department of Health and Human Services paints a more grim picture — up to 1.9 million deaths in the U.S., with about $200 billion in initial economic costs.

While researchers and public officials may only guess the possibility of a new influenza pandemic, many of the worst-case scenario forecasts for a current pandemic are focused on the 1918 influenza pandemic, which killed 675,000 people in the United States (nearly 0.8 percent of the 1910 population) and 40 million people worldwide from the early spring of 1918 via late spring of 1919.

In all recorded history, it is believed that only the Black Death that occurred throughout Europe from 1348-1351 destroyed more people (around 60 million) over the same period. The years 1918 and 1919 were not only problematic owing to the influenza pandemic; both years have represented the height of U.S. participation in World War I. Considering the severity and intensity of both the influenza pandemic and the First World War, quantities of work should be anticipated on the economic impact of each occurrence. While there is extensive literature on the economic implications of World War I, the spectrum of study into the economic impact of the influenza pandemic of 1918 is at best scarce. Some work has focused on the health and economic effects of pandemic victim descendants and the social class-wide disparity in mortality.

Perhaps an event that triggered 40 million deaths globally in a year will be studied carefully not just for its historical

57

importance, but also about what we might know about the tragic possibility of another influenza pandemic being faced by the nation. This chapter explores some of the economic consequences of the United States influenza pandemic of 1918. Chapter 1st segment introduces and addresses population disparities in pandemic mortality. Were deaths more severe in towns than in rural areas? Did fatalities vary according to race? Were the losses separate in terms of income? Detailed statistics on influenza mortality at the height of the pandemic are accessible at different regional and demographic rates. The inclusion of multiple mortality data series makes for an almost infinite amount of similarities and analyzes that provide the user with the ability to review the relevant data and produce his analyzes and conclusions besides those provided here.

Evidence of the impact of the pandemic on company and trade were collected from journal accounts written after the pandemic, with much of the stories found in publications from Little Rock, Ark, and Memphis, Tenn, the Eighth Federal Reserve District towns. Due to the almost total lack of economic data from this period, revenue, jobs, revenues, and wages, newspaper articles from the Fall of 1918 was used.

The lack of data, especially at the local level (e.g., city and county), is a possible cause for the absence of economic analysis on the subject. Still, some reports that have utilized accessible economic data are examined here and supplement the details collected from newspaper articles nicely.

Since the influenza pandemic happened in a world that was much different than today nearly 90 years ago, the scant economic statistics and more easily accessible mortality statistics at the period of the outbreak should be used to draw rational inferences regarding the economic and social effects of a modern-day pandemic. Despite advancements in medical technologies and expanded health coverage in the 20th century, fatalities from a modern-day influenza pandemic are still likely to be associated with race, income, and place of residence. Thus, the regional and demographic disparities in pandemic mortality from 1918 will shed light on the possible consequences of a modern-day pandemic.

## OVERVIEW OF THE IMPACT ON THE AMERICAN SOCIO-ECONOMY

In the United States, the influenza pandemic took place in three stages during the years 1918 and 1919. The first surge began in March 1918 and proceeded during the summer of 1918. The most destructive second and third waves happened in the fall of 1918 and in the spring of 1919 (the second being the worst). According to one researcher: "Spanish influenza traveled through the United States in the same manner as the colonists did, because it pursued their paths which had been railroaded... the pandemic spread along the axes from Massachusetts to Virginia ... the Appalachians leaped... positioned along the inland waterways ... it leaped straight through the plains and the Rockies to Los Angeles, San Francisco, and Seattle. Then, with stable bases on both coasts took time to spill through every space and corner of America. "But the effect of the pandemic on populations and regions around the world wasn't consistent. Pennsylvania, Maryland, and Colorado, for example, have the highest death rates, although they have almost little in common with these states. Arguments have been created that death levels in later-hit areas have been lower as authorities in certain areas have taken measures to mitigate imminent influenza, such as shutting schools and churches and banning travel. The influenza virulence weakens with time as normal influenza, and influenza that hit the West Coast was much slower when it reached the East Coast. Yet these explanations can not entirely justify why some towns and areas have suffered massive mortality rates while others have hardly been affected by the flu.

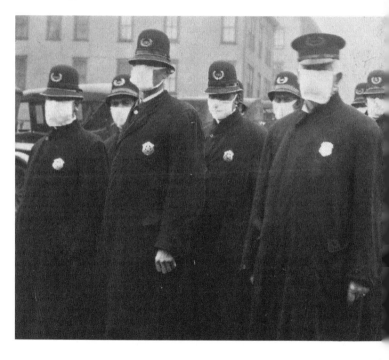

A lot of research has been conducted in the past few decades to provide information on why the pandemic has had such significant impacts on various parts of the world. World War I intensified the worldwide impact and scope of the pandemic, which is believed to have destroyed about 10

million people and 9 million troops in its way. The rapid influx of soldiers from across the world not only contributed to the outbreak of the epidemic, but hundreds of thousands of Allied and Central Power troops died as a consequence of the influenza pandemic rather than war. While battling deaths in World War 1 raised mortality rates for participating nations; civil mortality levels were much higher from the 1918 influenza pandemic.

In the United States, figures of combat-related fatalities from the influenza pandemic of 1918 are about one-tenth of those of civilian casualties. Typical influenza death rates continue to be the highest in the very young and the very elderly. What made the influenza special in 1918 was that death levels were the strongest for the population division aged between 18 and 40, and more so for males than females in this age range. Death was not usually triggered by the influenza virus itself, rather an immunological response of the body to the infection. People with the best immune systems were more likely to die than those with weakened immune systems.

One study estimates that approximately 49 percent of the 272,500 male influenza deaths in 1918 occurred between 20 and 39 years of age, while just 18 percent were under 5 years of age, and 13 percent were over 50. The fact that influenza struck the hardest males aged 18 to 40 has significant economic implications for the households who had lost their main breadwinner. As mentioned later in the study, the substantial loss of workers of prime working-age has had economic implications for the industry.

Given the magnitude of the pandemic, it is fair to claim that the 1918 epidemic was almost ignored in American memory as a catastrophic incident, which is wrong because learning from previous pandemics will be the best way to train fairly for potential pandemics. Many reasons can clarify why the

1918 influenza pandemic has not taken on a significant position in the history of the United States. First, the pandemic emerged around the same time as World War I. Despite their working circumstances and near interaction with increasingly mobile forces, influenza hit soldiers hardly. Secondly, most of the day's coverage centered on combat activities abroad and America's existing troop position. Therefore, the pandemic and World War I are viewed more as one event instead of two different ones. Thirdly, day-to-day illnesses such as measles, smallpox, and syphilis were incurable, and a lifelong feature of society. In comparison, influenza spread into towns, ravaged citizens, and vanished. Eventually, unlike measles and smallpox, no prominent citizens of that period died of influenza; therefore, there was no general belief that the epidemic was not harmless except to the socially influential, wealthy, and famous.

While the 1918 influenza pandemic may be an occurrence confined to the depths of American memory, the epidemic has had major economic consequences. Considering the non-zero probability of a potential influenza pandemic, the fact that most of these results were fairly short-lived will not render them less important to research. Though not a primary subject of this study, the 1918 influenza pandemic culminated in considerable human tragedy in selected regions, when the body counts overwhelmed the city and hospital (partially compounded by the absences of war personnel). For certain towns, such as Philadelphia, close to medieval in Europe during Black Death, corpses lie in the streets and morgues for days. Given the possible economic instability and human misery, recognizing the reaction of the state and federal government to the pandemic of 1918 can also offer some guidance about what the policy might do at some level to deter or mitigate a modern-day pandemic.

# MORTALITY DURING THE EPIDEMIC

Officially, in May 1918 to June 1919, 165,024 people were killed from influenza in Spain during the three outbreak waves. During 1918, mortality increased compared with mortality levels in the non-epidemic years. It may be concluded that this increased death was triggered by the influenza virus, specifically or indirectly. Nevertheless, as we strive for a cautious calculation, only deaths attributed to factors specifically related to an outbreak with such characteristics have been estimated. The most substantial changes were reported in respiratory conditions, possibly attributed to variations in standards where the diagnosis was made.

Influenza has caused significant increases in mortality among the seriously sick (chronic bronchitis, pneumonia, and pulmonary disease), the elderly (decline), and the very young (diarrhea and congenital weaknesses). In the absence of any other established trigger, we will conclude that the virus was indeed responsible for the increase in deaths due to 'other diseases.' The estimated number of 257,082 dead, indicating that 12 per thousand of Spanish suffered as a consequence of the outbreak. The high number of fatalities is remarkable and may be contrasted with other historical population disasters – the 237,000 casualties of the 1853–5 cholera outbreak, and the 345,000 fatalities incurred between 1936–9 during the Spanish Civil War.

Throughout Spain, as in the rest of the world, the 1918–19 pandemic triggered an unprecedented rate of mortality among the various age groups. Death levels in other influenza pandemics (e.g., in 1957 and 1968–9) were the highest among infants (0–1 year of age) and the older population (over 60 years of age), but the lowest mortality rates for young adults (20–40 years) occurred in 1918. The difference is striking between mortality in a non-epidemic year like

1917 and 1918. In 1917, influenza deaths clustered, as predicted, in the two most susceptible age classes, whereas in 1918, the highest numbers of deaths were reported in young adults aged 25 to 39. Mortality in the age classes that directly accompanied and followed these (20–24 and 40–44) was both quite high.

The second age group most impacted by the pandemic is children younger than one year old. This must be recalled that, in the first decades of the century, child mortality in Spain was quite high. Ultimately, child mortality rates increased by only 20 percent in 1918 over those observed in 1917.

# MORTALITY EFFECT OF THE PANDEMIC IN THE UNITED STATES

Mortality results from the influenza pandemic of 1918 can be contained in Mortality Estimates, a statistical study issued by the United States.

Survey: Survey Mortalities arising from hundreds of death causes are reported (depending on data collection level) and are often broken down by age, ethnicity, and sex in certain instances. Data are available at regional, local, and municipal level, and may be accessible every week, month, and year. In terms of scope, "(a)all death statistics are focused on overall fatalities, including fatalities of non-, deaths in hospitals and schools, and deaths of troops, sailors and marines."16 The mortality figures included in this analysis reflect deaths from both influenza and pneumonia in a single year as" it is not considered possible to research influenza separately and the different causes of pneumonia separately. That's because the U.S. Census collected the mortality statistics over time from a field of registration composed of an increasing number of states. Therefore, the mortality statistics are not reliably valid overtime for some nations. Regarding the reasons here, statistics on influenza mortality for the 1910s are valid for approximately 30 states that represent around 79.5 percent of the U.S. population on average. A glance at the states that recorded mortality information and did not do so does not show any systemic variations in population, wealth, and ethnicity across each community of states. Therefore, the mortality estimates available are unlikely to provide a skewed image of influenza mortality.

## ECONOMIC EFFECT OF THE FLU

This section of the book sheds light on certain economic consequences of the 1918 influenza pandemic. The main drawback of researching the economic impact of influenza in 1918 is the lack of economic evidence, as stated earlier. Several research reports utilized existing evidence to look at the economic impact of the pandemic, although these reports

71

are checked later. Nevertheless, despite the general scarcity of statistical evidence, the print media are a surviving source of knowledge on (some) the economic consequences of the 1918 pandemic.

For information on the impact of the influenza pandemic in these areas, newspapers in the Eighth Federal Reserve District areas of Little Rock and Memphis, which were distributed in the fall of 1918 is investigated. The accumulation of anecdotal reports from different communities combined will give a fairly clear description of the overall pandemic impact.

These general effects of 1918 can be used to extrapolate to the possible economic impact of a modern- pandemic. The 1918 Influenza pandemic in the Press segment provides reports and summaries of stories written in two Eighth Federal Reserve District City newspapers: the Arkansas

Gazette (Little Rock) and The Commercial Appeal (Memphis). In these publications and other journals (St. Louis and Louisville, for example), stories reporting the amount of sick or dead from influenza occurred almost regularly. Documents on the closings of hospitals, colleges, and theatres, as well as questionable treatments and solutions for influenza, feature regularly.

For the period 1914 to 1919, one research paper examines the immediate (short-) impact of influenza mortality on industrial incomes in U.S. towns. The paper's testable hypothesis is that influenza death significantly affected income levels in the industrial industry in U.S. cities and states before and shortly following the influenza of 1918.

The theory is focused on a basic labor market economic model: a reduction in the supply of manufacturing jobs arising from influenza mortality should have had the initial impact of decreasing the availability of manufacturing labor, raising the total labor and capital income per worker, and thereby rising real salaries. Labor immobility across communities and states is likely to have stopped state- wage equalization in the near run, so a switch away from comparatively more costly labor for capital is unlikely to have taken effect.

The empirical results support the hypothesis: In the era of 1914 to 1919, cities and states with higher influenza mortality witnessed a larger rise in wage growth for manufacturing. Another research used a common approach to analyze State wage development for the decade after the influenza pandemic. The writers claim in their unpublished paper that during the pandemic, countries that witnessed smaller amounts of influenza deaths per population should have seen better growth levels in per population revenue. Essentially, states with higher influenza mortality levels should have seen a greater cost gain per staff, and thus production per staff and higher wages after the pandemic. Using estimates of personal income at the state level for 1919- and 1930, the authors consider a favorable and statistically meaningful association between statewide mortality levels for influenza and subsequent per capita income rise.

The long- effect of influenza in 1918 was discussed in a recent study. The author questions whether influenza exposure in utero later in their lives have negative economic consequences for individuals. The research came about after the scientist studied data showing that pregnant mothers subjected to influenza in 1918 gave birth to infants that later in life developed significant medical conditions, such as epilepsy, diabetes, and stroke. The theory of the author is that the health endowment of a person is positively related to his human capital and productivity, and thus to wages and income.

Using decennial census data from 1960-, the author observed that populations in utero had decreased educational achievement after the 1918 pandemic, higher levels of physical illness, and lower wages. Specifically, whether they had been in utero during the pandemic, "men and women display significant and discontinuous declines in educational attainment. Children with tainted mothers were less likely to graduate from high school by up to 15 percent, while men's incomes were 5- percent smaller.

Most of the evidence indicates that the influenza pandemic of 1918 had short- consequences. Many companies, especially those in the service and entertainment industries, experienced double- sales losses. Many businesses that specialized in health care products experienced a revenue increase.

Some academic research suggests that the influenza pandemic of 1918 created a lack of labor, resulting in higher incomes (at least temporarily) for employees. Still, there is no good evidence that this gain outweighed the costs of the enormous loss of life and increased economic growth. Evidence also indicates that the influenza of 1918 triggered human resource losses among these in utero people during the pandemic, thereby creating consequences among economic development that happened decades after the pandemic.

## SOME DEMOGRAPHIC CONSEQUENCES

The most noticeable effect of the 1918–19 pandemic was the incredible death toll it caused. This disrupted a 3-year stretch of falling mortality rate in Spain. And from a demographer, the implications go deeper than that. It is therefore important to take into consideration the marriages that were not held, and the children who were never born. Since the turn of the century, in Spain, the regular period of marriage rates had a clear continuity. Autumn was the season of farming and also the period that several young people wed.

It is not surprising, then, that there was a slight decline in marriages during 1918. Yet widows gathered up the pieces a year apart and met a new partner. While not all are linked to the impact of the disease, there was a dramatic increase in marriages over the next five years, particularly among widows, indicative of human resilience.

It can be seen that the pandemic of 1918 proved to have little impact on the birth rate; on the opposite, a small uptick has occurred. The explanation for this resides in the seasonality of marriages and births, though, the largest rise in birth levels usually occurred in January and February, accompanied by a small spike throughout the summer. The babies that were raised in 1918 were conceived before the May outbreak arose. Even while the disease had little impact on the number of births that happened in 1918, it had a major negative influence on the number of conceptions that year.

Consequently, the birth rate fell dramatically in 1919. Nevertheless, birth rates increased during subsequent years, until 1923, despite the increase in marriage rates.

The outbreak was so deadly that it produced the largest annual natural increase deficit (4.0 percent) in the past two centuries in 1918. This has exceeded the shortfall of 1885, the year of the last cholera outbreak (1.7%), and that of 1939, the worst year in the Spanish Civil War (2.0%). Indeed, the community healed in the span of a few years, but the children born after the pandemic years belong to a depleted generation. They were born to parents who were both part of 'tiny' generations, humiliated by the 1885 cholera outbreak and the 1898 Cuban- Conflict. Furthermore, it seems that babies born in the preceding year of the pandemic or after the pandemic were more prone to suffer within their first 15 years of life than anyone because of the sequels of the infection.43 It was exactly the unlucky age that was, in effect, ravaged by the Spanish Civil War.

## LONG-TERM CONSEQUENCES AND MEMORIES

The influenza pandemic has had significant long-term effects in areas of Africa, while citizens do not talk about the epidemic directly in oral histories. The pandemic in southwest Tanzania reported maybe 10 percent of the population and ended in the worst famine documented in oral history. People equate the drought with the First World War, fought in the area from the 1914 German East Africa / Nyasaland frontier battles to the last pillaging until the German retreat in November 1918. As the first quotes demonstrate, people equate hunger with the disease too. That people call specific illnesses, rather than influenza, may contribute to the impression that illness was incidental to the famine and subsequent developments. However, it was the peculiarity of the 1918–19 influenza (high youth morbidity and mortality rates) and its timing, both in the annual rhythm period (planting season) and in combination with social and political upheavals – that contributed to famine and the reactions of citizens. This chapter explains how such responses in ethnography and indirect rule from the 1920s influenced the creation of a 'tribe.'

Historians and anthropologists learn about the Nyakyusa at the northern end about Lake Nyasa primarily from Monica and Godfrey Wilson's ethnographic work, undertaken between 1934 and 1938.4 Currently, the Nyakyusa is one of the main ethnic groups in Tanzania, comprising around 800,000 citizens. Nevertheless, the Wilsons initially suggested fieldwork among the 'Konde,' the common connection between Europeans during the 1920s and people in the region. Such people asserted citizenship at a finer level than the European- 'Konde' referring to the names of holy groves where chiefs sacrificed for rain and seed productivity, the names of mothers of specific leaders or long- founding leaders, the names of ancestral homes and the names of regions or villages.

A relatively small number of such people speak 'Nyakyusa' themselves. To suggest past links, the Wilsons understood cultural parallels around the area. Therefore, while they separated Tanganyika's Nyakyusa from the Ngonde in Nyasaland, they placed the communities of Kisi, Kukwe, Lugulu, Mwamba, Ndali, Nyakyusa proper, Penja, Saku, Selya, and Sukwa among the Nyakyusa. Core to the criterion for a 'men' by Monica Wilson was practice, 'for a while, the specifics beliefs and behaviors conveyed remain the same.' The age-, lines, and chiefdoms of Nyakyusa were merged as people drew from a collective whole for individual ceremonial performances.

Wilson believed that informants of Nyakyusa had a mutual understanding of ritual; although individuals received idiosyncratic explanations, 'it was at least a subconscious of Nyakyusa, and the meaning is political.' Therefore, 'the principles of a community (as opposed to those of individuals) are revealed' in individual ritual acts.

Defining 'tributes' by cultural and linguistic variables mirrored the British imperial attempts to create indirect control elsewhere in Africa. Throughout 1916, assuming possession over this portion over German East Africa, the British learned about the citizens of 'Konde,' a tradition of missionaries who had come from regions populated by Ngonde populations. Throughout 1926, under eleven chiefs and two dominant leaders, the British lumped much of the region's inhabitants into the Nyakyusa and Kukwe 'tribes.' Within the colonial system, designated chiefs contested for authority; those who were not named sought to dismiss others who were, while others fought or protested regarding the supreme position.

Many people opposed obedience to leaders with whom they had no existing ties of service and campaigned for different tribal concepts. In 1935, in favor of a council of leaders, the government abolished dominant leaders and redefined 'Kukwe' as 'Nyakyusa.' Unlike the ethnographers, the colonial logic of governance involved specific practices about their cultures and the traditional positions of rulers. To Europeans, the political system of Nyakyusa meant leaders of mutual descent, whose traditional practices included rainmakers (usually male kin) who provided protection and fertility for the group.

The district's first British officials followed practices that soothed the tensions accompanying the influenza pandemic. The 'corms drought,' a common term for oral history crises, culminated in two forms of response: those guided by households and those driven by individual leaders. State officers seldom observed reactions from families, though bosses acknowledged the extremely observable behavior.

Also, responses from leaders formed the partnership between the British and their people and defined the direction of indirect rule in part. Among other effects, by codifying the position of a supposed mainly class and its rainmakers as the defense of human health and land fertility, government and colonial ethnographers removed woman healers/officers from leading positions in community health and fertility and helped create one of the largest ethnic groups in colonial Tanganyika.

## THE CRISES

By 1917, in conquered south-west German East Africa, the conflict had convulsed many facets of civil and political activity. The Germans had hired porters and troops and had captured provisions and animals. The fighting took place all over the landscape. The British occupation of 1916 saw more requisitioning from other areas by a rising European empire and African powers. Originally, the British distrusted local citizens who had clear connections with German priests, who were removed by the Uk, and the Nazi government, the remains of which remained at large. The British expected anti-European uprisings such as those in Nyasaland, Northern Rhodesia, and Portuguese East Africa, but saw only tiny assemblies over thousands of years.

Many Africans were faithful to the Germans and supported the British. Some were imprisoned, some executcd. Some were happy to be rid of the Germans, such as some merchants and leaders who wished to achieve influence over the British.

In 1917 the British began raising duties, including crops required to feed soldiers in the war and using German logbooks to name leaders. They named those who had previously held no overarching right to govern and some who they viewed as German allies did not accept or exclude from official roles. And they 'sent in' leader Mwaikambo because he had supported them, even though under the Germans he did not hold such a position. Similarly, it was claimed that through the 'coming out' ceremony (ubusoka), Mwakalobo was not a chief but that Chief Mwakalukwa and his followers had offered him a role. In Selya, the British wrote as principal in Mwaipopo; Mwaipopo did not learn any German, so he was subordinate to Mwaihojo, who understood German and was not 'printed down.'

Through oral history, people also identified the British arriving in 1916 with diseases, particularly smallpox, and so academics connected famines with smallpox in Eastern

Africa between 1916 and 1920. Instead of inducing malnutrition, smallpox most often led to or worsened hunger conditions. Smallpox had been around for decades in eastern Africa, with small epidemics occurring through the mid-1920s. Epidemics and intense social contacts prevailed in dry seasons. Throughout the fighting, the thousands of troops who entered the area brought mutating smallpox variants into villages. During the dry season in mid-1917, as the war stopped, citizens assembled for funerals, dances, and feasts that allow smallpox spread quickly.

Most sources find the trek across the area by the German-led powers in October and early November 1918 to be a push to Northern Rhodesia rather than a major moment in the history of Southwest German East Africa. While the German-led forces left Portuguese East Africa with low rations, an officer among them reported, 'We had good times again in the region of Bena-Langenburg where the cattle herds supplied us with

meat and where both the sick and the well could collect milk.'
'Good times,' of course, indicated that they came to greater
food stores in the agricultural-rich areas of the eastern and
northern Si.

Several African porters and soldiers were scattered as the
German forces moved through the area. Some were from the
city, but unquestionably many were only trying to avoid
battle, starvation, and disease. Deserters dispersed to villages
where people were planting crops and expecting the season's
accompanying starvation and hard labor. Ironically, deserting
troops and porters who had survived smallpox in military
camps and tested German field doctors 'vaccines brought
viruses to their sanctuary, creating epidemic conditions.
Several thousand people continued with German- forces, and
they and the pursuing British forces were engaged in the' bulk
acquisition of local African livestock. Pillaging was a serious

blow to farmers who had been well trained for the planting in the rainy season.

It was during this pillage of October and November 1918 that the second wave of Spanish influenza rapidly spread, whose full impact was felt in December, struck down tens of thousands of people. Maybe 10 percent of the population — predominantly young adults — perished in a few months. As a result, eager planting did not satisfy the advent of rain, because millions of the populace laid sick, and many dead.

The important job of weeding could not be accomplished for those who planted when whole families were suffering from the flu, which resulted in the most serious drought in the oral history of the last century. In December and January, the district administration became ill-equipped to deal with influenza and suspended research for six weeks.

David Patterson said the influenza pandemic 'was almost definitely the single biggest short-term population tragedy in the history of [Africa].' Alfred Crosby noticed how the 1918–19 influenza varied from others: 'One, in a time of comparable length in world history, it destroyed more people than any other epidemic. Two, it destroyed an unprecedentedly high percentage of the leaders of a population who, according to reports before and since, would have avoided it without much damage. 'Influenza destroyed significant quantities of individuals between the ages of 20 and 40 everywhere it hit. This mortality pattern is significantly different from that of previous influenza epidemics in which the very young and the very old perished.

Through November 1918, the disease was prevalent on the northern end of Lake Nyasa. It first appeared by Indian Ocean trade in Eastern Africa: Mombasa by September 23, Portuguese East Africa by October 20 and Nyasaland by

November 5 in the south. The illness had traveled from Kenya to Uganda on the railway line late in October. Yet, since August, the German-led powers in Portuguese East Africa had suffered from what their physicians described as 'epidemic croup pneumonia.'

Therefore, the outbreak of the flu in the southwestern districts of British-occupied and German East Africa could have arisen from southern and eastern convergence, which had made the Nyasa-Tanganyika area a kind of 'disease corridor.'

The influenza death toll is almost impossible to estimate, even in the well-recorded regions accurately. Patterson claimed, based on little evidence, that at least 100,000 people died in the pandemic in Nyasaland and Tanganyika. To add to the elevated mortality risk, rehabilitation produced post-flu exhaustion that may persist for weeks or months, marked by emotional apathy, insomnia, subnormal body temperatures,

92

and low blood pressure. Such post-flu events would have ravaged farming communities that were urgently in need of planting and sorting, and that had already endured substantial losses to the competent populous.

The pandemic carried complex local perceptions, beginning with allegations of magic and witchcraft. TunyasyeIkofu remembered that at this period, many friends of her mother had died, perpetrators of witchcraft. The acting political district director, Major Wells, noticed escalated witchcraft-related crime and livestock stealing, which he linked to the pandemic. He also reported that the chiefs called for poison ordeals to classify the witchcraft practitioners. People soon understood the outbreak as an ikigwaja, a widespread plague. In the 1990s, KilekeMwakibinga, who escaped influenza, recounted that an ikigwaja tried to help his sister and aunt escape to Selya. Many people blamed the Irish for the outbreak, others for the war in general.

Faced with an ikigwaja, people worked with healers/officers to protect their kin. As the ikigwaja was tenacious, some chiefs called for meetings where they provided advice on the infection and steps to deter it. People viewed diseases as the consequence of their actions, so the relatives and chiefs, headmen, and healers at mass meetings tried to decide the guilty party.

Many nobles introduced a radical funeral- policy. Funerals were sad times but still opportunities for the vast amount of popular feasts and ceremonies, music, courting, flirting, battling, feasting, and chatting. A lot of sacrifice and feasting was geared towards the ancestors and the dead, but also towards the living, with whom debt ties were continually renegotiated.

Inability to adequately conduct a funeral, inability to alert family, dance, wail, pledge, and feast, all ensured even-

sickness and endangered crops. Hence the move to forgo public funerals was a drastic measure.

A man called Kalume told anthropologist Godfrey Wilson in 1936 about a shift in burial customs in Kukwe and Penja during an epidemic. Villagers were generally obligated to dig graves, but with fear of contagious illness, only immediate family treated a body. Kalume clarified that the specific disease they dreaded was one which 'killed the citizens badly.'

Kalume asked if this implied magic, 'yes indeed.' Chiefs halting funerals also given a display of unmistakable importance to modern European patrons. People have articulated social affiliation and differentiation by burials since pre-colonial times. The ability to stifle the show of difference enabled British officials to see important sameness around the country and see leaders as a class who governed what, in reality, were different activities in the field. The funeral and sacrifice moratorium prohibited largesse and shared feasting though at the same time concentrating on the chiefs.

## THE FAMINE AND LOCAL RESPONSES

The 'corm famine' that accompanied the flu lasted two years, which went mostly unrecorded in policy reports. The word 'corms famine' comes from the usage by women of banana corms as subsistence food to sustain their children. Local efforts against hunger fall into two groups, those managed by households and those including chiefs. Households, where they experienced the most acute effects, became the sources of first responses. People called for healer/officers (usually women) and used established tools and networks to manipulate. On the other side, the chiefs sacrificed their rainmakers and called on international male healers/officers to handle their villages, although there was no unified ethnic solution to the crisis across the north end of the lake. No working, united ethnic group existed, no dominant leaders, no focus on shared roots.

Chiefs took actions that were witnessed beyond the villages by significant historical players, including the British, who were capturing African traditions and political structure. Chiefs generated duties by bringing in the poor and feeding citizens who served them. Boys hoed up the bridewealth for rulers in return for livestock. There were two other practice collections conducted by other leaders.

One set of rituals was esoteric sacrifices to chiefly ancestors performed in sacred groves by rainmakers of chiefs and international healers/officers. These sacrifices had been prohibited by the Germans, partially fearing a revival of anticolonial sentiment, but after the British arrived, 'we go [and sacrifice] at daytime.' Drawing on ancient ceremonial partnerships and the reputation of individual healers/officers, chiefs and their headmen sacrificed to their ancestors to eradicate hunger. The villagers were barely interested in such mystical practices, most of whom neither saw the foreign healer/officers nor understood the specifics of the offers. Though chatter during these sacrifices was dense, they were done in locations most people never went to.

Esoteric sacrifices concerned individual chiefs and their ancestors, emphasizing the control of a chief over a region, the chief as embodying the land and its fertility by ancestral relations, and the relationships of the chief with distant and influential healer/officers. Several leaders in diverse areas pointed together to other fathers and god- founding figures. To outsiders, including the anthropologists 15 years later, mystic sacrifices highlighted certain commonalities and came to be seen as charter ceremonies that bound the chiefs 'people into a cohesive tribal unit. In contrast, chiefs specifically claimed that such sacrifices were not about tribal cohesion and that various chiefs had their sacrifices.

The second set of rituals sponsored by chiefs did not emphasize sameness among various chiefs but emphasized the relationships between an individual chief and his community and the duty of a chief to provide for local crop fertility. Chiefs also hired international healers/officers to treat the ground, buildings, forests, and banana plants in years of drought or sickness.

Treating the land sometimes coincided with esoteric sacrifices, but the two practices were interpreted differently by people in the villages, and the practices have various repercussions. Treatment of the soil took place in the homes and fields of the inhabitants, not in holy groves. Treating the land, commonly conducted during the 'famine of corms,' was an experienced exclusively to the local people, not involving leaders of larger communities with names such as Saku, Nyakyusa, Kukwe, or those who associated with a chief's sacred grove. Yet for Western listeners too, handling the ground became intangible.

People remember their houses rattling as medicines were splashed by healers/officiants, and reacting violently with fear and surprise despite the warning. Headmen and healer/officers told citizens to go inside and not come out, not to mess with the ceremony, to remain calm. Villagers nights were shaken by healer/officers who hurried around splashing drugs, shaking citizens out of sleep or night- talks, ignoring orders to remain quiet. People have, in certain instances, donated to charging the healer/officers. After all, the care for the soil was aimed at its ancestors to add prosperity to the soil. Such offers to ancestors were regarded by men, this splashing of medication on homes, banana trees, livestock, and vegetables, are so good that memories still exaggerate the effectiveness.

Headmen and chiefs obtained healer/officiants to treat the land at the people's request, and care of the land was not addressed exclusively to the chiefs 'ancestors. Leonard Mwaisumo, one of the study assistants of Wilsons in the 1930s, said that by treating the land, international healers/officiants "send the ancestors something, so they don't come up and trouble the country."

# CHAPTER THREE

# GOVERNMENT AND THE PEOPLE'S REACTION

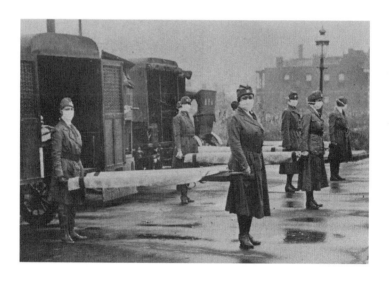

Public Health Departments' responses in Europe and the United States reflected the concepts that are common in culture and the science community. While much of the interventions were deeply rooted in the latest scientific principles, they could still be traced back to the Medieval and also Classical Plague and Pestilence periods. The notion of contagion causing quarantine and separation had its roots in the Justinian Plague. During the 19th century, epidemiological research by Snow and others furthered similar conceptions of communication contagion and comprehension. Because of these innovations and the confidence in man's capacity to manipulate behavior, public health departments develop. In the late 19th century, sanitation, vaccine campaigns and other public hygiene measures allowed agents of the public health to acquire influence and authority.

Nevertheless, the 1918-19 influenza pandemic overwhelmed public health authorities. The high morbidities arising from the severe influenza epidemic is both unexplained and frightening. Many of the interventions historically proven to function have been unsuccessful. They weren't equipped for an incident of this scale, missing the organization and resources and being limited by battle. And the great war produced the language of imperialism required to promote such authoritative reactions and sacrifices of independence.

## Authoritative measures

The public health authorities of both the United States and Europe have taken drastic steps to monitor Bubonic Plague epidemics going back to the medieval period. They managed to minimize pathogen transmission by preventing contact. They presented their public health directives in theoretical theories on their perception of how the influenza microbe transmitted across the air by coughing and sneezing, and their development of influenza pathogenesis. Because they believed that the pathogen was spread through the air, attempts were coordinated to monitor contagion and discourage anyone affected from breathing the same air as the uninfected. Public meetings and individuals getting together in tight proximity have been used as a possible disease-transmitting mechanism. Public health officials claimed that adequate airflow and fresh air were "the strongest of all general preventive strategies, and this means preventing mass gatherings," which converted into the divisive yet necessary step of shutting certain public buildings and banning public meetings during the outbreak.

The rigidity of these laws differed tremendously with the strength of the local health authorities and the severity of the outbreak of influenza. In the United States, the American Public Health Association (APHA) Committee proposed measures to restrict large-scale gatherings in a survey. The committee held that assembly of people was dangerous, with combining bodies and exchanging air in cramped spaces. Non-essential gatherings had to be excluded. Because these were needless gatherings, these decided that saloons, dance halls, and cinemas would be closed, and public funerals should be banned. Churches were authorized to stay active, but the committee was of the view that only minimal services could be provided, and intimacy should be reduced. Road cars with inadequate ventilation, crowding, and uncleanliness are considered to be a particular danger to the population. The committee welcomed the staggered opening and closing hours of shops and warehouses to reduce overcrowding and allow citizens to stroll to work where they possibly could. Many of Britain's rules were milder, such as restricting appearances in the music hall to fewer than three consecutive hours and calling for a half-hour rest in events. Theatres, cinemas, festivals, and shooting competitions were all stopped in Switzerland as the outbreak struck, contributing to a state of emergency. This variability in the reaction was most likely due to variations in public health department authority and social recognition as expected of their initiatives. This took a common interest in the idea of contagion, and some confidence in science's behavior to help them to conquer this epidemic.

The most widely addressed and debated measure of public safety in publication journals was the closure of schools. The severity of the disease in Britain contributed to the closing of the public elementary schools. In France, students with any symptoms will be removed from school and their siblings. If three-fourths of the students were missing, the whole class would be suspended for fifteen days. Many felt closing schools was a good tool for preventing illness, but argued that it always came too late when most students and teachers were ill. The closing of the school was not as generally known in the United States. JAMA reported that "the desirability of closing schools in a big community amid an outbreak is a calculation of questionable interest." The APHA Committee has discussed its importance, challenging the efficacy toward the lack of educational quality. In fact, school suspensions were considered to be less effective by large metropolitan metropolises than in rural centers where the school served the infectious agent's point of propagation. It was not widely accepted that schools and other public facilities would be closed as public health measures to the popular epidemic. One editorial in the BMJ notes that "every vulnerable urban citizen will, sooner or later, contract influenza whatever public health authorities may do; and that the more schools and public gatherings are suspended, and the community's general existence dislocated, the greater would be homelessness and poverty." Such steps involved a compromise of human rights for the benefit of humanity, which thereby demanded a powerful public health authority. Both the Departments of Illinois and New York State Education recommended that patients be quarantined before all clinical symptoms of the illness subsided. We believed that the danger of the influenza outbreak was so serious that protection for the individual was necessary. In their study, the APHA committee leaders decided that influenza cases would be placed in isolation. Due to the strain on facilities, only severe cases needed to be treated when those with minor influenza had to remain at home. The APHA has sponsored voluntary quarantines in institutions such as asylums and schools, to shield citizens from the outside environment. For the several combat training centers set up in the United States to equip troops for war, the use of administrative quarantines was extended. These camps were prime targets of major influenza epidemics, with waves of people from all over the world. When sick, the people were held in complete confinement, with regular quarantine in whole villages. Such steps were quickly enforced in such camps where people had already dedicated themselves to their nation and government power.

## Preventative measures

The Committee of the American Public Health Association (APHA) released a study detailing effective means of stopping the spread of the epidemic and minimizing its severity. They first noticed that the disease was incredibly contagious and "produced mainly by discharges from sick people's nose and throats." They tried to avoid transmission through disrupting contact networks, such as sputum drainage droplet contamination. They claimed the infection was induced by hand contact and eating utensils. They, therefore, called for legislation to prohibit specific cups from being used and to control coughing and sneezing. They decided to implement respiratory health awareness campaigns and advertising about the risks of hacking, sneezing, and reckless handling of nasal discharges. They tried to educate people on the importance of hand-washing before eating and the advantages of general hygiene. Departments of Public Health have released Flu Posters to warn the population and to reduce virus transmission. The representatives also indicated that the response would differ based on nature and living circumstances of the population. Measures will be targeted to remote or urban regions, with coordinated management to promote mandatory monitoring and case evaluation.

In their suggestions to reduce the spread of the illness and prevent disease, public health authorities extended the concepts of infection to hygiene methods and consideration for ventilation. They held the well ventilated, airy rooms the fostered wellness. Preventative strategies focused on the same propagation theories and illness germ theory. Similar concepts were brought into effect in hospitals when separate influenza wards were established for influenza victims, and the number of beds per ward was decreased to limit the disease spread. Some with conditions of pneumonia had been isolated from the others to keep the majority from progressing to a more dangerous state. In small, closed quarters, sheets were placed between the beds to imitate isolation and provide a cubicle for each patient. Neither patient was permitted to leave their bed until they had been 48 hours free of fever. Soldiers were told to feed 5 feet apart in the mess-halls in the military camps. Sleeping in the head to foot was often introduced to reduce air room sharing. One camp used these preventive strategies by airflow and spoke about their success. They believed that their raging influenza outbreak stopped because people were shut out of sunshine in the field, airy halls, and prevented from gathering together.

One primary preventive factor was the method of disinfection and sterilization. The practical preventive recommendations used the latest discoveries of the need antiseptic conditions, created by Lister and others. All bedding and rooms were to be disinfected regularly to destroy whatever pathogen impregnated them. It was done in naval ambulance trains by wiping down the train with a mild antiseptic izal solution. The sputum created was to be destroyed and thought to be contaminated with the microbe. The sputum cups were cleaned and disinfected twice daily at one hospital, while nasal discharges were collected in paper napkins. An antiseptic hand solution was conveniently positioned at the

influenza ward for those in service. One French report also indicated that the influenza ward workers would wear blouses inside the ward and remove them on departure. Such preventive disinfection procedures used scientific theories of the theory of bacteria to reduce transmission.

Another form of prevention was the gauze mask, incorporating common ideas in contagion and germ theory. Throughout the United States, it has been generally adopted by health care professionals for use in clinics. The face masks were a half-yard gauze, wrapped like a triangular bandage that protected the lips, nose, and ear. Such gauze covers also served to avoid the removal of the contagious droplets from the mouth and from the paws, infected with a microbe, from being inserted into the mouth. The hand barrier was judged to be more critical than the air barrier. For certain countries, the general public was still carrying the mask. In San Francisco, a court law declared the gauze masks a necessity of the local city. It was also extended to January to cover San Diego. This rhyme has become a common way to recall ordinance to citizens.

They found that wearing masks contributed to "a significant decrease in the number of influenza cases." However, a test in the Great Lakes showed no such advantageous effects. Mask wearing by hospital corps had little impact on disease occurrence as 8 percent who used the mask were infected when only 7.75 percent of non-mask wearers were infected. The masks were widely used by others in an attempt to prevent the pandemic influenza disease, despite these results.

## Prophylaxis

APHA committee leaders have also discussed strategies to improve natural tolerance to the disease. They said he would prevent emotional and physical fatigue. Residents were allowed to get good rest, fresh air, and general grooming. The

French Study also recommended the prevention of over-fatigue and cold weather. The Royal College of Physicians voiced this view suggesting that wearing warm clothes outside would protect the body from sweating. They also believed that a healthy diet and drink nourishment are beneficial, stating that calm and over-exertion have bad effects. "Unlike prevention interventions, these methodologies do not appear to have a clear empirical foundation. Rather, they represent traditional social, philosophical leanings wellbeing and the potential to combat infection. Thus to a degree, the medical and public health officials were still using common sense notions to combat this new infectious terror.

However, one form of avoiding infection was scientific, more complex, and more controversial. This was gargling and rinsing of antiseptic solution out of the nasopharynx. Physicians believed that it made sense to disinfect the nose and mouth to avoid contamination because the disease was spread through the upper respiratory passages. Another approach was to gargle with chlorinated soda, combined with warm water. Dr. F. W. Alexander advised that electrolyte disinfect fluid by gargling and sniffing through the nose as a mouthwash for influenza. Others gargled and rubbed the nasopharynx with a mild carbolic acid solution and mixed the drug with quinine to avoid infection. Dr. James Bach recommended a more effective way of cleansing and disinfecting the nasal gaps and upper air passages. He favored a boric acid solution and sodium bicarbonate mix. The substance was to be sprayed into the nose and would then melt, causing mucus release to flush the membranes through osmotic action. This approach has a theoretical foundation but no empirical proof of the efficacy. They as well try some of the drugs that were developed to prevent influenza, which focused on medical theories but not empirical evidence.

APHA members claimed gargling had little value as they cleared the barrier of infection from the protective mucus.

Committee members of the American Public Health Association agreed on the only approach to prevent infection was by using vaccines. Vaccines may prevent or mitigate influenza infection and the sometimes lethal complications of the disease induced by the influenza bacillus or streptococci and pneumococci strains. They felt the latest vaccines in development would be tested and distributed because they were effective in preventing infection. The committee recommended testing the experimental vaccines on susceptibles with similar subjects and controls and using appropriate scientific methods. They admitted that the source of the influenza was unknown and that an effective vaccine has little "scientific basis." Many public health authorities shared their views of the influenza disease's with the scientific and medical community regarding its origins.

## HOW U.S. CITIES TRIED TO HALT THE SPREAD OF THE 1918 SPANISH FLU

The devastating second wave of Spanish flu arrived at America's shores in the late summer of 1918. Carried by doughboys coming home from Europe after World War I, the increasingly virulent influenza first traveled from Massachusetts to New York and Philadelphia before heading west to strike terrified cities of St. Louis to San Francisco.

Lack of a vaccine or even an established source of the epidemic left the mayors and town health authorities no choice than to improvise. Will the classrooms be locked, and all public hearings banned? Would they need every person to wear a face mask with a gauze? And would it be unpatriotic to close down essential financial hubs in times of war?

The Spanish flu destroyed approximately 675,000 Americans and a staggering 20 to 50 million people globally before it was all over. Many U.S. towns suffered much worse than most, though about a century later, there is proof that the early and well-organized reactions delayed the transmission of the disease — at least temporarily — while communities that lost their foot or lowered their guards paid a heavier price.

## Philadelphia Parade

By mid-September, the Spanish flu spread like flames across Philadelphia's army and naval facilities. Still, Wilmer Krusen, Philadelphia's chief of public safety, told the nation that the affected soldiers suffered merely from the old-fashioned seasonal flu and that it would be contained before infecting people.

When the first few civilian reports were identified on September 21, local doctors feared that this could be the start of an outbreak, but Krusen and his medical board suggested that by remaining warm, holding their feet dry and their "bowels free" Philadelphians might lower their chance of contracting the flu, writes John M. Barry in The Great Influenza: The Saga of the Deadliest Pandemic in History

While the levels of civilian infections rising hourly, Krusen refused to cancel the forthcoming Liberty Loan parade scheduled for September 28. Barry notes that infectious disease authorities advised Krusen that the parade, which was supposed to draw several hundred of thousand Philadelphians, would be "a ready-made flammable medium for a conflagration." Krusen argued that the procession would proceed, as it would collect millions of dollars in war funds, so he played down the possibility of transmitting the disease. A patriotic parade of veterans, boy scouts, marching bands and civic dignitaries marched 2 miles across central Philadelphia with spectator-packed sidewalks on September 28.

Only 72 hours after the event, all 31 hospitals in Philadelphia were packed, and at the end of the week, 2600 people were dead.

George Dehner, author of Global Flu and You: A History of Influenza, claims that although Krusen's plan to stage the parade was certainly a "poor one," the incidence of infection in Philadelphia was rising by the end of September only. "The Liberty Loan parade undoubtedly poured fuel on the flames," says Dehner, "but it was still going along very nicely." (How St. Louis Flattened the Infection Curve) The approach to public safety in St. Louis couldn't have been more specific. Just before the region had confirmed the first case of Spanish flu, health chief Dr. Max Starkloff put area physicians on high alert and penned an editorial in the St.

Louis Post-Dispatch about the significance of reducing crowds.

After a flu epidemic first erupted through the general populace of St. Louis at a local military base, Starkloff spent little time closing the colleges, locking down movie theatres and pool rooms, and prohibiting any public meetings. Company owners had pushback, but Starkloff and the mayor kept their position. As illnesses swelled as predicted, a network of local nurses tended to thousands of ill people at home.

Dehner claims public health authorities in St. Louis were willing to "flatten the curve" to prevent the flu outbreak from spreading immediately as it did in Philadelphia because of such measures.

"In such a short amount of time, it's the swarm of new cases that overwhelms the capability of a community," says Dehner. "It magnifies any issues you may have." The highest incidence rate in St. Louis was just one-eighth of Philadelphia's death rate at its lowest, according to a 2007 study of Spanish flu data. This is not to suggest St. Louis escaped the unharmed outbreak. Dehner says the Spanish flu's third outbreak, which emerged in the late winter and spring of 1919, struck the midwestern city hard.

## San Francisco Enforces Wearing Of Masks

Health officials in San Francisco put their full confidence into the gauze masks. Governor William Stephens of California proclaimed it was the "patriotic obligation of any American citizen" to wear a mask, and finally became the norm in San Francisco. Citizens found without a mask or inappropriately displaying one in public were arrested, charged with "disturbing order," and fined $5.

Jacobs says in his book that the gauze masks reported by city officials were "99 percent evidence against influenza" were, in fact, hardly effective. The relatively low infection rates of San Francisco in October are possibly attributed to well-organized campaigns to quarantine all naval installations until the flu struck, as well as early attempts to close schools, ban social gatherings and close all "public amusement" locations. On November 21, a whistle blast indicated that San Franciscans might eventually take off their masks and the San Francisco Endemic. Believing masks is what first protected them, retailers and theatre managers pushed back against demands receiving from the public. As a result, San Francisco wound up having some of the strongest Spanish flu mortality rates nationally. The 2007 report showed that it might have decreased fatalities by 90 percent if San Francisco had kept all of its anti-flu protections in effect until the spring of 1919.

## HOW OREGON REACTED TO THE 1918 SPANISH FLU PANDEMIC

"Beware of sneezers and coughers!"Read the Oregon Journal's evening edition on 5 Oct. It was a night out on Saturday. A lot of people had intentions to head to the movies. And it was raining. Fall had arrived in Portland, bringing the normal cold and flu season with it. But starting now, the newspaper reported that anybody who sneezed or coughed in a public theatre should be promptly asked to leave.

The unexpected law was a precaution against the spreading of a new flu virus throughout the United States, the article clarified. It then reassured Oregon had not yet seen any cases. This was not true.

Just two days before the first case of the new lethal disease had arrived.

That was the year 1918. The First World War went on in Europe mixed with the battlefield headlines came reports of a growing wave of sickness. Where the epidemic emerged was unknown, but because Spanish newspapers, uncensored during the war, were the first to report this increasing health problem, it was quickly called "the Spanish flu."

The Spanish influenza pandemic has been one of the most lethal in history. It affected as much as one of every four human beings in the world, contributing to approximately 50–100 million deaths. The pandemic destroyed more lives than World War I — and in less time.

Currently, the virus has been classified by scientists as a new influenza strain H1N1. Like in the latest novel coronavirus pandemic, the word "novel" implies that people were never subjected to it. So because citizens have no previous experience, they did not have any tolerance to it.

Since Portland was afflicted by the Spanish flu more than a century ago, so how Portlanders responded has an eerie connection to what we are seeing.

In Portland, a private soldier, on his way to Texas for training, became the first reported case at Portland. He'd been good that day. He remained sick the following day and headed to Portland City Hospital. Diagnosed with Spanish flu, he was assigned to medical quarantine.

The signs begin with a cough, close to severe flu. Unlike the telltale spots of measles or smallpox, there were no visible symptoms of illness.

The upper respiratory system has taken control of Spanish flu, a form of influenza virus. Unlike today's coronavirus, it triggered respiratory problems. It dispersed almost invisibly, equally, through the airborne droplets of coughs and sneezes.

As the sickness intensified, so did the pain. Patients would cough blood from a shortage of oxygen and start turning blue. A lethal form of pneumonia settled in and caused uncontrollable hemorrhaging that filled the lungs, leaving victims drowning in their blood.

Young children and the elderly were more likely to be exposed, but what was disconcerting about this new strain of flu virus was how it generally affected safe adults, particularly those in their 20s and 30s.

This was the same demographic as the troops sent in the First World War to serve in Europe. As such, the disease spread quickly among troops who were housed in barracks and troops nearby.

Benson Polytechnic School's rectangular, two-story brick structure in northeast Portland was a recruiting base for 300 cadets during the war. It became the epicenter of the epidemic when four confirmed Spanish flu cases were recorded. The building was lockdown instantly.

Medical director George Parrish, of Portland, got to work. He launched a registry of public locations, including schools, churches, and streetcars, to identify as "no sneeze" areas. "Individuals would be cautious not to sneeze, cough, or transmit illness germs anywhere on packed buses," he added. He has invited area pastors to help convey Sunday's letter.

The Morning Oregonian announced that Parrish was "confident that protective steps and residents' implementation of appropriate procedures would help to mitigate the outbreak." Seattle had already been affected by the virus. At least a dozen deaths have already been reported. The mayor of Seattle outlawed street gatherings and told residents not to meet in churches.

The nation's capital also started its shutdown in Washington, D.C. The White House, the Supreme Court, and Capitol Hill locked their doors to the general public.

The Red Cross mobilized its branches worldwide. It dedicated its supply of hospital materials to the cause and demanded that all nurses register and be trained.

The surgeon general ordered all state health officers to shutter amusement schools and locations, and to cancel all public meetings anywhere the virus was detected.

## Spread the word, not the virus

Parrish launched a public awareness program in Portland. He approached theatre owners and told them to show slides in front of movies to warn viewers to cover their sneezes. He encouraged teachers to ventilate classes and educate their pupils about influenza prevention and diagnosis.

School assemblies and gym classes were stopped as a precautionary measure. But there was no clear way to know the degree of which the virus had spread across the region. Had they found it in time? Might this only be handled by isolating the soldiers? No-one knew for sure, but Portlanders felt hopeful at the moment.

"With the few cases that have so far been confirmed here, there appears to be a reason for urgent intervention," said Mayor George Baker, of Portland.

## Wash hands, social distance

Just a week after Portland's first case of Spanish flu, the Oregon State Health Board required all public meeting areas to be shut down nationwide. Parades were stopped, Churches also discontinued their programs, Restaurants left bare. Silent dance-halls. And all of a sudden, 36,000 students from Portland have nowhere to go.

In addition to the closures, stores, and businesses limited the hours of work. The famous department store of Portland, Meier & Frank, requested consumers not to come into their shop but to put delivery orders instead. Officials advised people of Portland to wash their hands and keep at least four steps apart — the concept of "internal distancing," Parrish said. "The condition is promising. The newspaper declared, "Significant Outbreak of Influenza Impossible." The newspaper confirmed the virus' first death in Portland three days later. By November 3, precisely one month after the first case reported at Portland — the death toll had risen to 227 in Portland. On the same day, 17 new cases were registered in Oregon City. Bend recorded 100 incidents and his first death. Hood River County registered 250 cases and called for those with nursing skills to support healthcare staff make house calls to patients who are home-bound.

That day, in Seattle, Seventeen people had died; the day before, nearly 2,000 new cases reached San Francisco in three days. They made it compulsory to wear a mask, punished by penalty, or incarceration.

The outbreak grew so quickly that it became extremely difficult to monitor. On Monday, Nov. 18, Portlanders woke up to rain again, picked up their newspaper and read what must have been a foreboding statistic: the number of Americans affected by influenza has already surpassed the number of American soldiers killed in the battle, calculated at 100,000.

But when they looked down at the day-to-day political cartoon, they noticed kids back in the classroom faking sneezes as an excuse to be dismissed.

"Flu ban is off," the caption read. "School starts today." Parrish, the Portland health official, also claimed that concentrating on those with coughs was the only approach to stop the virus. If you're tired, he said, remain home. It is classified as a felony catching a cold in general.

But Portlanders gradually ignored the threats and went back to daily life. They began riding the streetcars again, heading to work and continue their vacation shopping.

Parrish could see, two months after the epidemic, that things were getting worse. Health authorities have been blaming the public for disregarding the recommendations. Portland had desperately wanted a new plan.

The mayor proposed an immediate measure to classify influenza formally as a "communicable disease," putting it alongside smallpox and scarlet fever. That will make the " stay at home" instructions constitutionally enforceable to those with the disease.

The mayor directed the police of Portland and the Multnomah Patrol to back up the health inspectors while doing their rounds.

The next week, the Oregon State Health Board updated the status of influenza, rendering it legally quarantinable in the county.

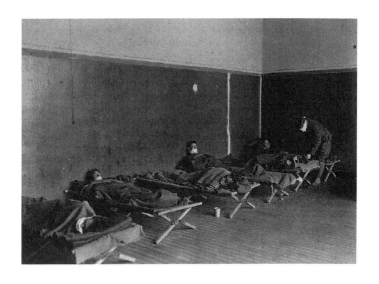

## Ringing in the New Year

As Portlanders made their resolutions and prayed for the New Year, there is no denying that most expected that the pandemic would soon let go of its grip on the city and leave. No day had elapsed in the three months after the epidemic started without an influenza-caused death.

Hospitals overflowed. Hundreds of new reports were also coming in. Behind the hospital entrance, officers stood to watch and prevent patients from joining, driving individuals away with minor health issues.

The epicenter of the first incidents, Benson Polytechnic School, was turned into a temporary hospital with 200 seats. Portland's mayor suggested doing what communities like San Francisco had done: require mask wear.

He imposed a $500 penalty (the equivalent of over $9,000 today) and 60 days in jail to anybody who refused to wear a mask in any public room, to show he was concerned.

Portland City Council discussed and vetoed the Mayor's legislation. Attorney W. and T. Vaughn found the forced wearing of masks "unconstitutional," claiming that politicians "tried to muzzle us like a herd of hydrophobic dogs."

## The ebb

Slowly, as January went on, the crisis started to wane. In Salem, removed the restriction on a public meeting, reopened schools and theatres, which were closed for many weeks. In Portland, some 7,000 doses of a new serum arrive. It was called Rosenow, named after a doctor who had created it in the Mayo Clinic. There was a pharmacy founded to provide free vaccinations.

At the end of January, Portland has been ravaged by the outbreak for nearly four months. Health authorities braced for a third storm. Although it tapered the number of new incidents. By February, the virus appeared to have run its course.

It had eventually claimed the lives of some 3,500 Oregonians. Though the day's general news was still bleak, Portlanders was able to breathe a little easier.

## THE PEOPLE'S PREVENTIVE MEASURES

People also used a variety of measures during the first half of the 20th century to seek to protect themselves from the flu. One of these was the camphor, or camphor trees, extracted from Cinnamomumcamphora. People might wear a bag of camphor around their necks to fend off the virus, while nurses and physicians might inject it with a hypodermic needle into an infectious patient's arms and legs. Today, camphor is one of Vicks VapoRub's main ingredients — though it is limited in lower and healthier doses by the Food and Drug Administration.

Other early flu precautions involved gargling saltwater, wearing masks, eating oranges, and—at least with one set of parents—warning people not to kiss their baby. These remain good ideas, but the CDC stresses that having a regular vaccine is one of the easiest strategies to avoid flu, particularly for those who still practice healthy flu season habits.

# CHAPTER FOUR

# VACCINES AGAINST THE FLU

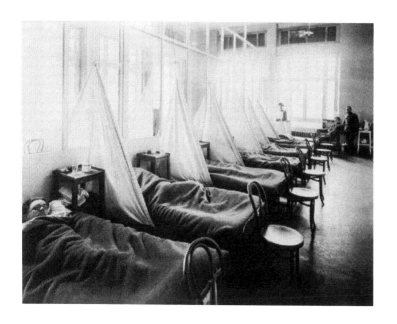

When people write about the 1918-19 Spanish Influenza pandemic, they typically begin with the staggering global death toll, the huge number of people infected with the pandemic virus, and the medical field's inability to do anything to treat those infected. Although these causes were hallmarks of the catastrophic event, doctors and health officials in the U.S. and Europe remained optimistic in creating vaccinations and immunizing hundreds of thousands of citizens in what amounted to be the largest-scale scientific trial. What vaccinations did they come up with? Have they done something to strengthen the immune system to avoid the epidemic from spreading?

Next, with the figures, the US population in 1918 peaked at 103.2 million. During the Spanish Influenza pandemic's three waves between Spring 1918 and Spring 1919, 200 out of every 1000 people contracted influenza (around 20.6 million). About 0.8 percent (164,800) and 3.1 percent (638,000) of those affected died secondary to influenza or pneumonia.

There were a few vaccinations available at the time to combat certain illnesses — smallpox vaccination had, of course, been used for more than 100 years; Louis Pasteur had created a post-exposure prophylaxis rabies vaccine after an experience with a wild animal; typhoid fever vaccinations were created. After the late 1800s, diphtheria antitoxin — a drug produced from the blood of previously contaminated animals — was used for treatment; an early version of a diphtheria vaccine was used, and experimental cholera vaccinations were developed. In 1911, Almroth Wright also studied a full-cell pneumococcal vaccine against gold miners in South Africa. Manufacturers have produced and sold various vaccines of limited value for mixed heat-killed bacterial stocks.

Not much was known at the moment in terms of understanding influenza as an infectious disease. Many medical practitioners believed influenza was a specific contagious illness that was introduced seasonally, typically in winter. And then, moderate forms of influenza remain hard to discern from other severe respiratory disorders without clear diagnostic devices. The devices of the period could identify only microbes, not tiny pathogens.

Yet physicians and scientists tried to understand how yearly influenza they were used to being linked to the rarely common and extremely infectious illness in years that we now recognize were influenza pandemics (1848-49 and 1889-90).

In an 1892 paper, German scientist Richard Pfeiffer (1858-1945) reported to have identified the causative agent of influenza — he mentioned rod-shaped bacilli present in each influenza case that he investigated. Nevertheless, by inducing the disease in laboratory specimens, he was not able to show Koch's postulates. However, other experts acknowledged his observations, and they believed Pfeiffer's influenza bacillus was responsible for seasonal influenza, as it was named.

But as the 1910s progressed and bacteriological approaches evolved, other researchers published results which were in contrast with the findings of Pfeiffer. He noticed his virus in stable persons and others suffering from diseases that were not influenza. Moreover, in influenza situations, they scanned for Pfeiffer's bacillus and, in certain situations, could not detect it at all. While several physicians assumed that Pfeiffer had diagnosed the perpetrator right, an increasing number of others had started to reconsider his results.

Those true believers had every incentive to expect that a vaccine could eliminate influenza when the epidemic started its second arrival in the early fall of 1918 in the United States. On 2 October 1918, William H. Park, MD, New York City Health Department head in bacteriologist, began consulting on the influenza vaccine using a Pfeiffer strain. The New York Times reported that Royal S. Copeland, New York City Health Commissioner, identified the vaccine as preventive against influenza and a "transfer of an old theory to a new illness." Park created his vaccine from Pfeiffer's heat-killed bacilli removed from ill persons and tested it on Health Department volunteers (New York Times, October 2, 1918). Three doses were delivered 48 hours apart. He reported in the New York Medical Journal by October 12 that he was vaccinating workers of army bases from major businesses and troops. He expected to provide proof in a few weeks to prove the vaccine's effectiveness (Park WH, 1918).

The Newark Evening News reported in November that 39,000 doses of the Leary-Park influenza vaccine had been packaged, and most doses had been used. (Timothy Leary was a researcher at the Tufts University School of Medicine.) While it was too early to say whether the vaccination was successful, "... the normal individual may not need to be fearful of the consequence of the vaccination. Neurotic and rheumatic patients, though, tend to be prone to the vaccine,

although infants receive it with less discomfort than adults"
(Newark Evening News, 1918).

By 13 December 1918, Copeland was not so confident about the vaccine for his department. He told the Times that it seemed that vaccinations produced from Pfeiffer's bacilli had little impact on influenza prevention. Instead, he was sure that E.C was producing a combination of bacterial vaccine (streptococcal, pneumococcal, staphylococcal, and Pfeiffer's bacilli). Rosenow had become an important preventive at the Mayo Base. And although he figured most citizens in New York were already vulnerable to Spanish influenza, he announced that he would help Park plan enough of the Rosenow vaccine to immunize people in New York all winter (New York Times, December 13, 1918). Just over 500,000 doses of the Rosenow vaccine have been created (Eyler, 2009).

The University of Pittsburgh, the University of Tulane, and some private scientists made their vaccinations. They also used the Convalescent serum (Boston Message, January 6, 1919; Robertson & Koehler, 1918). On December 14, 1918, the Deseret (UT) Evening News reported that free vaccination had been distributed in communities around the state.

Based on my survey of the publication newspaper and medical journal papers, it is evident that during the pandemic years, hundreds of thousands, if not a million or more, of vaccine doses were made.

The American Journal of Public Health's Editorial Committee sought to place a damper on people's perceptions of the vaccinations. They reported in January 1919 that the new influenza causative agent was still uncertain and that the vaccinations being developed had only one possibility of being aimed against the correct target. They stated that secondary infection vaccinations make some sense, but much of the vaccine being developed must be considered as experimental. Recognizing the rather ad hoc production of the nature vaccine in the present situation, they recommended that test groups be used for all the vaccines and that the discrepancies between test and experimental community be reduced as to the probability of infection, duration of infection during the outbreak, and so on (American Journal of Public Health Editorial Committee, 1919).

Certainly, none of the vaccines mentioned above-avoided illness with infectious influenza – we already recognize that influenza is triggered by a virus, and none of the vaccinations shielded against it. But were some of the bacterial infections that evolved secondarily to influenza protective? Vaccinologist Stanley A. Plotkin, MD, claims they didn't. He told us, "The bacterial vaccinations produced for Spanish influenza were possibly unsuccessful because pneumococcal bacteria were not reported to exist in many serotypes and the bacterial group they called B at the time. In other terms, the vaccine pioneers could not classify, distinguish, and manufacture all the possible disease-causing strains of bacteria that were circulating at the moment. Indeed today's children's pneumococcal vaccination protects against 13 of the bacteria's serotypes, and the adult vaccine protects against 23 serotypes.

However, a 2010 article describes a meta-analysis of 1918-19 bacterial vaccine trials, which proposes a more positive view. Based on the 13 reports that mcct inclusion requirements, the authors suggest that the attack risk of pneumonia following seasonal influenza infection could have been decreased by some of the vaccinations. We claim that vaccination may have contributed to cross-protection against several associated pathogens, given the small number of strains of bacteria in the vaccines (Chien, 2010).

Finally, in the 1930s, researchers discovered that influenza was primarily triggered by a virus, not a bacterium. Throughout the result, Pfeiffer's influenza bacillus will be renamed Haemophilus influenzae, the term that preserves the tradition of its long-standing, albeit misleading, influenza affiliation. And now, vaccinations for pneumonia-as well as H. Form B influenza vaccinations – are commonly accessible for disease prevention.

## Vaccine Development across the United States

Physicians at the Naval Hospital on League Island, Pennsylvania (the Philadelphia Naval Shipyard) described their approach to a vaccine: "In the concept of a drowning person grabbing a straw, a stock influenza vaccine was used as a preventive in fifty specific cases and as a curative agent in fifty other uncomplicated cases" (Dever 1919). We made a B-made vaccine: pneumococcus, Streptococcus, Staphylococcus, and Micrococcus catarrhalis (now Moraxella catarrhalis) influenza and varieties. For a four-dose treatment, a growing dosage contained between 100,000,000 and 200,000,000 bacteria per cubic centimeter. The inspectors confirmed that no vaccinated person (who were medical workers) were ill but also stated that stringent safety precautions, such as the usage of helmets, gloves, and so on, were provided. None acquired pneumonia, but one experienced pleurisy (lung lining infection) in a sample of sick patients treated therapeutically with the vaccine. They reported, "The duration of the disease [in those therapeutically treated] ... was certainly reduced, and prostration seemed to be less severe. The patients that were not helped were those that were admitted four to seven days after their illness began. This was out of all proportion with the number of emerging cases of pneumonia and the extent of the control cases infection. The outcomes were also more striking; the sooner the vaccination was delivered. "Eventually, they concluded that," The number of patients infected with vaccines and the number immunized with it is entirely too small to allow any deductions; yet to the degree that no adverse findings follow their usage, it would seem certainly healthy and perhaps desirable to suggest their usage. We report that Spanish influenza did not hit San Francisco until 1 October 1918 and that thus the personnel at the training station had time to take protective steps (Minaker 1919). Due to the position of the base on Alameda Island, isolation was convenient, reachable only by boat from San Francisco and Oakland. Naval Yard staff were allowed to use a regular spray of antiseptic to the throat.

Beyond these interventions, the writers acknowledged that "actions were taken to develop a prophylactic vaccine," while there was a "huge difference of opinion about the pandemic's exciting origin." Pneumococcus and streptococcus, in general, are seen as the source of the most severe complications. We have wanted to achieve a society of B, in the middle of opposition. Rockefeller Center influenza with a catastrophic event should be used in the vaccine. Generally, the vaccination contained B. Influenzae, 5 billion bacteria; Types I and II pneumococcus, 3 billion each; Type III pneumococcus, 1 billion; and Streptococcus hemolytic (S. pyogenes), 100 million.

To assess toxicity, Guinea pigs were first injected with the vaccine and then inoculated five volunteer lab workers. Labor experiments confirmed that their count of white cells decreased, and their scra agglutinated B. Influenzae (meaning they had antibodies that responded to the bacteria in their blood). Local swelling and discomfort caused side effects from the injection but no abscesses. They were authorized to continue, further vaccinations were planned, and 11,179

154

civilians and soldiers were inoculated, some at Marc Island (Vallejo, CA) and San Pedro, as well as civilians affiliated with the Naval Training Station in San Francisco. The prevalence of influenza cases was lower in most experimental groups than in the uninoculated groups (although no detail is available about how the data were obtained for the uninoculated groups, nor is there detail about how a case was defined). Patients who were inoculated got the shots only three weeks after influenza in California emerged, and it's difficult to know whether they had already been treated and infected. The percentage of influenza cases in control groups varied between 1.5 percent to 33.8 percent (the latter were nurses in San Francisco hospitals). In comparison, others in the inoculation community were sick with influenza between 1.4 percent and 3.5 percent (the latter were medical corpsmen on service in an influenza ward).

Another use of the vaccine was documented at the Puget Sound Navy Yard (Ely 1919) in Washington County. Police reported that when a party of sailors came from Philadelphia, influenza entered the Navy Yard (it's uncertain precisely when they came, although the report notes that "the investigation duration was from September 17 to October 18, 1918"). In total, a streptococcal vaccine has vaccinated 4,212 men. The authors estimated that the prevalence of influenza attacks ranged from 2% to 57% in the vaccinated and from 1.8% to 19.6% in the unvaccinated. They noticed, however, that there were no deaths among the vaccinated people. They said, "We agree that the use of killed cultures as mentioned stopped the progression of the disease in many of our workers and changed its favorable course in others." Influenzae did not take part in the outbreak.

E. C. Rosenow (Mayo Clinic) confirmed the use of a combined bacterial vaccine in Rochester, Minnesota, where, in his original research, about 21,000 residents obtained three doses of vaccine. He reported that "In inoculated, the overall occurrence of identifiable influenza, pneumonia, and encephalitis is around one-third as high as in the uninoculated community. In the inoculated, as in the uninoculated, the overall mortality risk from influenza or pneumonia is just one-fourth as high. "He will move on developing his vaccine in about 100,000 men."

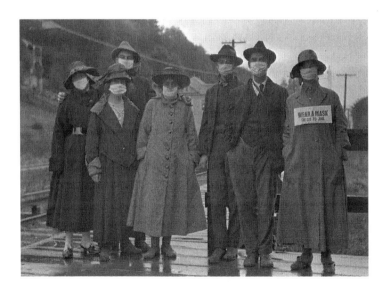

In an editorial titled "Prophylactic Inoculation Against Influenza," the American Association of Medicine Editors 'Journal cautioned that "the evidence collected is clearly too insufficient to make a professional assessment on the efficacy of the vaccinations." In particular, they answered Rosenow's paper: "To define just one example: the situation of a hospital of Rochester — where fourteen nurses (out of how many?) contracted influenza about two days (how much earlier?) of the first vaccination (at what point in the epidemic?), and only one disease (out of how many possibilities?) eventually emerged over six weeks — may be duplicated. In other terms, when all the cards are on the table until we recognize all the reasons that might potentially affect the outcomes as much as possible, we can not provide a fair basis for evaluating whether or not the effects of prophylactic influenza inoculation justify the interpretation they have received in some quarters.

## Measuring Success

Certainly, none of the vaccines described above-prevented infection of viral influenza – we now know that influenza is caused by a virus, and none of the vaccines protected against it. But were any of the bacterial infections that developed secondary to influenza protective? Vaccinologist Stanley A. Plotkin, MD, claims they didn't. He told us, "The bacterial vaccinations produced for Spanish influenza were possibly unsuccessful because pneumococcal bacteria were not reported to exist in many serotypes and the bacterial community they called B at the time. In other terms, the vaccine researchers could not classify, distinguish, and manufacture all possible bacterial disease-causing strains. Indeed today's children's pneumococcal vaccination protects against 13 of the bacteria's serotypes, and the adult vaccination protects against 23 serotypes.

However, a 2010 article describes a meta- of 1918- bacterial vaccine trials, which proposes a more positive view. Based on the 13 reports that meet inclusion requirements, the authors suggest that the attack risk of pneumonia following seasonal influenza infection could have been decreased by some of the vaccinations. They reported that vaccination might have contributed to cross-protection against several associated strains, given the small number of bacterial strains in the vaccinations (Chien 2010).

It wasn't until the 1930's did researchers establish that influenza was caused by a virus, not a bacterium. Eventually, Pfeiffer's influenza bacillus would be called Haemophilus influenzae, the term that retains the legacy of its long-standing, though inaccurate. And today, vaccines for influenza-as well as H. Type B influenza vaccines – are widely available for disease prevention.

# THE STATE OF SCIENCE, MICROBIOLOGY, AND VACCINES CIRCA 1918

The influenza pandemic of 1918–1919 significantly altered the biomedical knowledge of the disease. At its creation, evidence gathered during the previous big pandemic of 1889–90, became the base of scientific understanding. Otto Leichtenstern's dissertation, first reported in 1896, identified the key epidemiological and pathological aspects of pandemic influenza and was frequently quoted over the next two decades. In 1892 and 1893, Richard Pfeiffer revealed he had found the origin of influenza. Pfeiffer's bacillus (Bacillus influenza) became a significant subject of concern between 1892 and 1920, with some confusion. During the great pandemic, the role played by that organism or such species in influenza dominated medical debate.

During the 1918–1919 pandemic, multiple vaccinations were created and used. The scientific literature was full of conflicting reports of their success; evidently, there was little agreement about how to interpret the recorded outcomes of such vaccine trials. The consequence of the vaccine dispute was both a further deterioration in faith in Pfeiffer's bacillus as an influenza agent and the introduction of a new collection of standards for appropriate vaccine research.

When the great influenza pandemic of 1918–1919 started, research undertaken after and directly after the previous pandemic, that of 1889–1990, were the most significant sources of information on infectious influenza. The influenza pandemic of 1889–90 was the first in the Western world to arise since the pandemic of 1848–49. That meant it was the first to occur after more affluent nation-states had been created, professional health departments and vital statistics programs, are the first to researched using modern pathology and bacteriology methods. The pandemic of 1889–90 created a rather significant literature production and two very critical biomedical syntheses. In 1891, Franklin Parsons, a director of the Medical Department of the Local Government Board in London, published a 300-page paper on the pandemic, focused on surveys of all sanitary districts in England and Wales and on local research in selected areas. Five years later, relying on continental, especially German, science, and clinical literature, Otto Leichtenstern published the definitive scientific literature.

These two major work particularly Leichtenstern's were well known from which American authors of medical textbooks and research plays, such as William Osler and Frederick Lord, would derive their findings and hypotheses during the next great pandemic over the next two decades and the criteria by which medical authority would evaluate them.

It means much regarding the primitive condition of influenza research in the early 1890s that the most significant and enduring finding of these two landmark works was that influenza was a particular illness, and contagious.

It spread very rapidly, quicker than any other known contagious disease, and it caused explosive local outbreaks. It never emerged naturally, however, nor did it fly quicker than flying through humans. Near analysis quickly dismissed reports of infections that arise without precedent cases or in areas that have no interaction with sick citizens. In comparison, scattered groups, such as those within jails in highly polluted areas, often escaped entirely. While influenza appeared most often during the winter and spring months, the pandemic spread in all latitudes in both hemispheres, at all human-inhabited altitudes, and in all temperatures. Overt climatic or environmental conditions didn't do it. A major influenza outbreak was never a single case. One or two further infections are sometimes accompanied by a large epidemic within months. Early 1890s, physicians acknowledged that it was difficult to treat influenza and that minor symptoms were often associated with other respiratory and catarrh-like diseases. Through clinical and epidemiological reports, they were very confident that the influenza of the great pandemic of 1889–90 was the same illness that had triggered the influenza pandemics in the past, including the one in 1848–49. The more vexing question was that this pandemic influenza was the same illness as the widely recognized influenza or grippe condition that existed almost every year. Parsons certainly felt they were distinct diseases; Leichtenstern accepted, though less assertively.

## INFLUENZA VACCINES

The existence of Pfeiffer's bacillus as the probable source of influenza is mirrored in the usage of vaccinations in the USA during the 1918–1919 pandemic. By 1918, the effective usage of other vaccinations, in particular those against rabies, typhoid fever, and diphtheria, as well as the use of anti-toxin diphtheria, had created strong hopes for an influenza vaccine. Those who already had a vaccine in their possession were soon off the mark to advertise their vaccinations as healthy prevention or influenza cures. Drugmakers have been actively selling temperature, influenza, and flu vaccinations in their stores. The structure of these vaccinations remained unknown. There were reports of market gouging and kickbacks as consumer fear and competition swelled.

Physicians such as M.J. have backed preexisting vaccinations of unknown composition. Exner, who vigorously advocated the vaccine produced some six years ago by his friend, Ellis Bonime, in media interviews and testimonials. Bonime was a late proponent of tuberculin treatment for tuberculosis and a promoter of the opsonin hypothesis of immune reaction and vaccination therapy. His vaccination was believed to eliminate diarrhea, measles, and blood poisoning. The boosterism of Exner has paid out some dividends. At least one town, Far Rockaway, New York, has confirmed it would supply all its citizens with the Bonime's vaccine.

Early in the pandemic, more respected and well-placed experts created vaccinations that were directly focused on Pfeiffer's bacillus. On October 2, 1918, the New York City Health Inspector, Royal S. Copeland, tried to convince people that aid was on the way as a vaccine was being created by the Health Department's chief of labs, William H. Park, which would protect against this dreaded disease.

The successes Park developed in these same laboratories in combating diphtheria with anti-toxins and vaccinations gave Copeland's announcement more weight. Park demonstrated to his colleagues that he and his team have repeatedly been able to distinguish Pfeiffer's bacillus from influenza outbreaks and that his laboratory had identified the new form, shown that animals injected with it developed strong antibodies, and produced a heat-killed vaccine to be delivered at two-day intervals in three doses.

Park's wasn't the only bacillus influenza vaccine Pfeiffer chose to make an early arrival during the pandemic. Timothy Leary, professor of bacteriology and pathology at Tufts Medical School in Boston, developed another Pfeiffer's bacillus vaccine. It was formed from three locally isolated strains, and heat-killed and treated chemically. Leary has been marketing his vaccine as both a prevention and an influenza drug.

OtherPfeiffer's bacillus vaccines soon followed. The University of Pittsburgh's Faculty of Medicine isolated 13 strains of the Pfeiffer's bacillus and produced a vaccine from them by changing Park's techniques. The creators of the

Pittsburgh vaccine separated their strains in the disaster environment of the pandemic, primed the vaccine, checked it for safety in several experimental animals and two individuals, and handed it over to the Red Cross for medical use — all within one week.

Charles W. Duval and William H. Harris, from the Department of Pathology and Bacteriology at Tulane University, created their own chemically destroyed bacillus vaccine for Pfeiffer in New Orleans. Their reason for its usage was the widespread existence of the bacillus in cases of influenza and the precedent of the typhoid vaccine, which they adopted in their administration plan.

It was not just the heads of bacteriological laboratories who acted on the assumption that Pfeiffer's bacillus was the source of influenza, and on that theory, they created vaccines. A few private physicians have achieved the same. Horace Greeley of

Brooklyn, New York, announced that 17 strains of the bacillus were collected from 17 people, and from these "strains," he developed a heat-killed vaccine designed to be delivered in three expanded doses. He immunized his doctors with it and gave eight liters to all colleagues who did the same.

These vaccines were used widely. Park's vaccine was released to both the military and private physicians for use in Army camps. This was often seen by industrial workers as a corporate policy, including the Consolidated Gas Company's 14,000 employees and the US's 275,000 employees in Steel Company. Leary's vaccine was widely utilized by certain private doctors in Northeastern state custodial facilities throughout the outbreak.

Duval and Harris reported about 5,000 people getting vaccinated, most of whom were workers of major New

Orleans companies. Nearly without question, all commenting on the usage of the bacillus vaccines from these Pfeiffer's reported success in avoiding influenza.

## THE FALTERING CASE FOR PFEIFFER 'S BACILLUS

The apparent success of these vaccines initially helped to boost trust in the function of Pfeiffer's bacillus. But there was also an accumulation of other data. They initially had their methodology and expertise challenged after experts reported difficulties in isolating Pfeiffer's bacillus from influenza cases.

But the evidence slowly mounted against Pfeiffer's bacillus, first ambiguously and then absolutely. J.J. Keegan, a naval medical officer, working in the Boston area, released an early study on studies conducted in the First Naval District over the two weeks between 28 August and 11 September 1918 during an outbreak of 2000 cases. Keegan made a special attempt to research the bacteriology of the epidemic. In all influenza events, he had trouble isolating Pfeiffer's bacillus from throat washings or sputum and patients admitted to hospital with other conditions and wondered whether the organism might be harbored in the sinuses or any other location that is more elusive. In 82.6 percent of 23 cases, as he resorted to lung punctures in postmortem life and lung cultures, he succeeded in isolating Pfeiffer's bacillus.

Other ambiguous results came from a future American influenza expert called Edwin Jordan. Jordan reported on a large bacteriological sample at the University of Chicago of patients infected with influenza and other illnesses before and during the outbreak. In his cases, he mentioned having no clear bacteriology. In both instances of influenza, no microorganism was found, while in 64 percent of influenza cases, he detected Pfeiffer's bacillus, and that was more prevalent than any other organism, its relative occurrence differed greatly among cases. He isolated B. Influenzae in colds and other infections of 14 percent.

A group of Cook County Hospital's medical staff in Chicago conducted a detailed analysis using 3,000 blood agar culture plates, and the protocols they carried would have found B influenza if there were any. They observed that in just a limited amount of cases, Pfeiffer's bacillus was present: in just 4 percent of crops produced from washed sputum samples and in just 8.7 percent of postmortem lung cultures. In the lungs of a soldier who had died of influenzal pneumonia, they discovered the organism in virtually pure nature. They found Pfeiffer's bacillus to be the source of the pneumonia outbreak. Throughout this study, they observed that pneumococci were the most widespread species isolated, occurring throughout 70 percent of sputum cultures and 38 percent of garnet swab cultures. Type IV pneumococci have been identified in 50% of autopsy-made lung cultures. Types I – III was all present at lesser frequencies as well.

Evidence ran stronger against Pfeiffer's bacillus by early 1919. In February, David Davis announced that he had succeeded in isolating what he described as B, utilizing specific morphological and cultural parameters. He reported Influenzae in only 8 percent of 62 influenza cases. As noted earlier, he has identified this organism in higher concentrations of measles, varicella, tuberculosis, and pertussis events. There was no chance, and he claimed that the bacillus Pfeiffer had become pathogenic to humans. For both forms of meningitis involving bronchopneumonia when B was removed from the spinal fluid. Influenza often occurred in a pure or nearly pure society. He suggested that whatever could be the origin of influenza, the most dangerous symptoms are attributed to secondary invaders, including streptococci, pneumococci, and B. influenza.

Similar conclusions were reached by Frederick Lord and colleagues in Boston. Lord had already isolated B, and so had Davis. Influenzae originating from diseases other than influenza. In this pandemic, he and his collaborators detected Pfeiffer's bacillus-like bacteria in 84 percent of 38 infected victims of influenza, but also in 41 percent of the throats of participants of the Harvard Students 'Army Training Corps, who had no record of illness over the previous three months. Lord concluded B. Influenzae could be regarded as part of the natural human throat flora. However, there was little confirmation as to whether the species present in usual throats and other diseases with common anatomy and culture and staining features were simply equivalent to those found in influenza.

A possibility remained, it seemed, that would explain recent bacteriological observations, and yet rescue a position for

Pfeiffer's bacillus in influenza etiology. Maybe there was a pseudo-influenza bacillus, or various strains of B, as the situation of diphtheria might show. Influenzae that didn't just cause influenza. In this case, discovering morphologically similar species to Pfeiffer's bacillus in certain diseases was not evidence against Pfeiffer's position in influenza.

Several researchers investigated this possibility by trying to form Pfeiffer's bacillus strains, but their findings did little to bolster faith in B. influenzae's role in influenza. H.F. Rapoport, a naval medical officer from Cambridge, Massachusetts, used the Antibodies B fastening check kit. Influenzae in convalescent sera from viral pneumonia and regular sera regulation. He reported that unique antibodies to Pfeiffer's bacillus were produced from influenza-accompanying pneumonia during convalescence but that these had poor complement-binding properties. He was unable to decide whether one or more strains of Pfeiffer's bacillus spread throughout the outbreak. However, he found that polyvalent antigens in his samples did not yield stronger results than monovalent ones.

Park and his associates studied cultures that were taken from 100 influenza cases. In certain instances, over centuries, traditions have been picked up twice, Careful clicking of antigens shows there was a broad range of B types. Influenzae, the bacteria collected from a human were very consistent over time, yet various forms were derived from specific individuals. Much like pneumococcus, he indicated that B. influenza over the years had altered into distinct forms in the throats of healthy carriers. In influenza cases, Pfeiffer's bacillus, he concluded, has to be considered a secondary invader.

# ALTERNATIVE ETIOLOGIES, OTHER VACCINES

Other things had been proposed during the pandemic as the cause of influenza, but these were disposed of quickly. Captain George Mathers, a medical officer of the Army who died of influenza during his research, identified and described a streptococcus that developed a green color on blood agar plates A Fort Mead, he extracted his green-producing streptococcus from 87 percent of cases of influenza and pneumonia. However, in only 58 percent of those cases, he was able to extract Pfeiffer's bacillus.

In the early months of the pandemic, the Mathers streptococcus was noticed. For starters, Jordan thoroughly checked for it in his research but found little facts to make it appear as a possible source than B. Influence. Then, studies in both Europe and America found the likelihood that influenza could be triggered by a filterable virus. (p. 148–9) The controversial finding that influenza could be induced in humans by inoculating content from the noses or throats of influenza patients that had gone through a bacterial spread was a problem. French and Japanese investigators confirmed this approach had worked in transmitting influenza.

Such observations were not verified by American researchers; Cook County Hospital researchers used this approach to inoculate seven human volunteers without inducing illness. They did the same with colonies produced from the samples of influenza pneumonia lungs, and with positive findings, they inoculated two Rhesus monkeys.

Specific laboratory and human inoculation experiments aimed at detecting a filterable virus were also negative. Such negative findings were also verified by extensive human experiments with influenza sponsored by the U.S. Navy and the U.S. Public Health Service.

As confidence in the role of Pfeiffer's influenza bacillus waned, the policy of vaccine prevention changed. Vaccines developed later in the pandemic — and almost all formed in the south of the country and on the West Coast — were delivered separately or in mixtures consisting of certain species. Vaccines have been gradually explained as avoiding influenza-accompanying pneumonia. A physician in Denver and the medical personnel at the Puget Sound Naval Yard developed killed streptococci vaccines. In Seattle, the latter was used by sailors and also by civilians.

Mixed vaccines have been more prevalent. These usually contained both streptococci and pneumococci. Sometimes, it also involved staphylococci, Pfeiffer's bacillus, and more newly infected, wild specimens in the ward or morgue. The vaccine produced by Edward C. Rosenow of the Division of

Experimental Bacteriology at the Mayo Clinic was the most commonly used, and traditionally the most interesting.

Rosenow concluded that the precise formulation of a vaccine meant to deter pneumonia than in use needed to suit the distribution of the lung-infecting microbes. Despite this cause, he claimed that his vaccine formulation always needed to be re-adjusted. His initial vaccination composed of killed bacteria in the following proportions: 30% pneumococcal forms I, II and III; 30% pneumococcal type IV and 'green-producing diplostreptococcus;' 20% hemolytic streptococcal; 10% staphylococcus aureus; and 10% B. Influence. Earlier, he removed Pfeiffer's bacillus. The Mayo Clinic extensive delivery of the Rosenow vaccine to physicians in the upper midwest. No one appears to say for sure how many individuals got this vaccine, but Rosenow obtained results on 93,000 people who received all three vaccines from doctors,

23,000 who received two vaccinations, and 27,000 who received one.

The vaccine by Rosenow has been widely distributed. The City of Chicago embraced it. More than 500,000 doses of the vaccine were developed by Chicago Health Department Laboratories. Most of that was allocated to doctors in Chicago, and the remainder was handed over for use in Illinois to the state health agency.

## THE PANDEMIC AND BIOMEDICAL KNOWLEDGE

Even though the experience of the great pandemic of 1918–1919 gave American medical experts a deeper understanding of the dangers of pandemic influenza. While allowing epidemiologists to expand the detailed knowledge obtained on influenza outbreaks, little had been accomplished to unlock the mysteries of the disease. The 1918–1919 experience served to de-construct existing biomedical knowledge.

This void in fundamental knowledge would not soon be filled. In 1927, when Jordan published his massive, 500-page authoritative synthesis of influenza literature, the most essential and important features of influenza were still unknown. Jordan advised his readers that influenza can only be identified by its occurrence pattern — its epidemiology. His origin was unclear, and his diagnosis was unknown.

This remained unclear if tolerance for influenza remained gained, and if so, how long this persisted. It was still unclear why pandemics occurred as they did, and why they spared some places. This was still unclear that influenza in isolated events and minor outbreaks that happened each year was the same disease that spread throughout the pandemics. He maintained the practice of separating "influenza" from the "epidemic influenza." Jordan indicated that it could be necessary to adjust the virulence of the then-unknown influenza agent and whether this agent might be filterable. However, in 1927 these were only speculations for which no clear proof was available.

In short, the three decades after Leichtenstern released his main synthesis have seen little addition to the fund of basic science information of influenza, following considerable attempts by researchers utilizing the best research tools available to them.

# CHAPTER FIVE

# HISTORICAL LESSONS

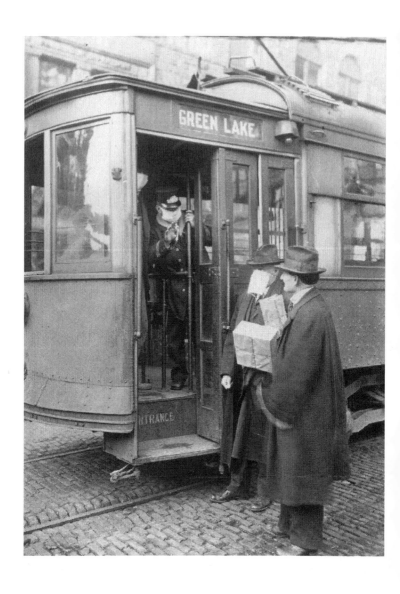

2018 marked the 100th anniversary of the influenza pandemic of 1918, which killed about 50 million people worldwide. The magnitude of this pandemic was triggered by a dynamic interplay of viral, host, and societal factors. Here we review the viral, genetic, and immune factors that led to the magnitude of the 1918 pandemic and addressed the implications for modern preparedness for the pandemic. We address unresolved concerns as to whether the H1N1 influenza virus of 1918 was more virulent than previous influenza pandemics, and why certain persons survived the pandemic of 1918, and others succumbed to it. Although current research indicates that viral factors such as haemagglutinin and pieces of the polymerase gene more likely led to a strong, dysregulated pro-inflammatory cytokine storm in pandemic patients, a change in case-fatality toward young adults in the 1918 pandemic was most likely associated with the host's immune status. For children and young adults, the absence of pre-existing virus-specific and

187

cross-reactive antibodies and cellular immunity undoubtedly led to the high attack intensity and widespread dissemination of the H1N1 virus in 1918.

In comparison, in the older (> 30 years) adult population, reduced mortality rates contribute to the positive impact of pre-existing cross-reactive immunity. In addition to the function of humoral and cellular immunity, an increasing array of evidence indicates that individual genetic variations concerning single-nucleotide polymorphisms (SNPs) lead to variations in the intensity of influenza virus infection. The frequency of influenza fever is often reported to cause co-infections of bacterial viruses, and probably measles and malaria, co-morbidities, malnutrition or obesity, which likely affected incidence, which results in H1N1 disease in 1918. Additionally, we also address the current problems that we will encounter in the sense of every potential influenza virus pandemic, such as increasing population dynamics, antibiotic resistance, and climate change. Over the past decade, the amount of dangerous influenza virus variants reaching the human community from animal reservoirs (including extremely pathogenic H7N9 and H5N1 viruses) has risen significantly. Therefore, an appreciation of previous influenza virus pandemics and the lessons we learned from them was never more important.

## Host Factors Associated with Influenza Morbidity and Mortality Variations in 1918

The influenza pandemic of 1918 is notable for its elevated morbidity and mortality levels. It is necessary to note that there have been major differences in mortality within and across countries (Mills, 1986; Johnson and Mueller, 2002; Johnson, 2006). General estimates assume an average mortality rate of 2.5–5 per 1,000 people worldwide. However, that may be a reasonable approximation for certain countries [e.g., Australia (2.8/1000), Austria (3/1000), Demark (4.1/1000)], it constitutes overestimation for certain countries [e.g., Argentina (1.2/1000), Uruguay (1.4/1000), American Samoa (0/1000)], and extreme underestimation for others [e.g., Nauru (160/1000), Western Samoa (236/1000), Cameroon (445/1000), such findings suggest that host conditions also had a significant impact on the outcome of the outbreak, in addition to viral factors.

## Age

The age of an individual played an important role in determining one's risk of death during the influenza pandemic of 1918. Typically, a "U" shaped curve is developed when seasonal influenza mortality rates are graphed against population age, as the maximum mortality occurs in the very young and the old. Pandemic outbreaks (to varying degrees), on the other hand, are distinguished by a change in case-fatality towards younger age groups. This was especially prevalent during the 1918 pandemic when young adults (15–30 years) experienced such a historical high mortality rate that a mortality curve shaped like "W" was made. The underlying mechanisms which cause this change in mortality are not fully understood but are likely to be correlated with the immune status of the host.

## Immunopathology

Traditionally, high mortality levels in young adults during the 1918 pandemic is due to the activation of an unusual, dysregulated pro-inflammatory reaction (often referred to as a 'cytokine storm'). The theory is based on laboratory experiments utilizing the replicated influenza virus of 1918 in specific animal models. Such laboratory experiments have demonstrated that the influenza virus of 1918 caused a strong, dysregulated pro-inflammatory reaction, possibly leading to the severe lung lesions found in victims of the influenza pandemic of 1918. However, this dysregulated immune response was also found in both the potentially pathogenic avian H5N1 virus and the 2009 pandemic influenza virus, both in normal and laboratory infections. It is important to remember, though, that all laboratory trials of the influenza virus of 1918 to date have been undertaken in immunologically naïve specimens. It is not generally representative of the human condition in 1918 because, before 1918, influenza outbreaks had triggered epidemics and pandemics. Therefore, it may be concluded that a significant proportion of the human populace in 1918 should have experienced at least one prior influenza virus outbreak, with the likely exception of remote countries/communities, culminating in pre-existing humoral and cellular immunity. Whether this pre-existing immunity would cross-react with the H1N1 virus of 1918 remains unknown, and if so, if it would boost or dampen any dysregulated pro-inflammatory reaction in young adults.

## Humoral Immune Response

Unlike young adults during the 1918 pandemic, older adults (aged 30–60 years) fared significantly better. This finding is likely to indicate the beneficial effects of the humoral immunity that preexists. Until 1889, when it was absorbed by an H3 influenza virus that triggered the so-called "Soviet" influenza pandemic (1889–92), it is theorized that an H1 or N1 influenza virus existed throughout the human community. Accordingly, individuals born before 1889 (i.e., all 30 years of age or older during the 1918 pandemic) should have developed cross-protective antibodies while those born after 1889 should have become immunologically resistant to the 1918 H1N1 pandemic virus. The lack of pre-existing influenza-specific or cross-reactive antibodies in children and young adults in 1918 undoubtedly led to the elevated attack incidence and rapid virus dissemination. Only those affected during the pandemic's first "season" phase developed a defensive immune response to the pandemic's second wave, more virulent, "weather" phase of 1918–19. Interestingly, unlike the bulk of the world's aged, aged communities in rural areas, including Indigenous Australians, Alaskan Natives, and Latin Americans, suffered elevated mortality during the 1918 pandemic. It most definitely illustrates the reality that the historic circulating influenza viruses that provided cross-protection were not introduced to such distant communities.

Conclusive evidence that protective influenza virus-specific responses to an antigen are still long-lived comes from the influenza pandemic of 2009. There, older people subjected to the influenza virus of 1918 (or its immediate descendant), 60–90 years before the 2009 pandemic, were shielded from infection and serious disease, because they retained the antibody reaction that cross-reacted with the 2009 pandemic strain.

Interestingly, a new report indicated that previously diagnosed people with influenza-like illness in the years before the 1918 pandemic (1916–1918) were likely at an increased risk of having clinically significant respiratory disease during the 1918 pandemic's autumn wave.

Likewise, the existence of cross-reactive but non-neutralizing antibodies has been correlated with immune complex deposition and increased severity of disease during the influenza pandemic of 2009. Such findings indicate that disease protection relies not just on the availability of pre-existing antibodies, but on their ability to neutralize the influenza virus strain involved.

## Cellular Immune Response

The issue of prior exposure to influenza virus in the general population before 1918 raises the question of why a pre-existing cellular immune response, particularly cross-reactive

CD8 + T cells, gave too little defense to young adults during the influenza pandemic of 1918?

A robust response to CD8 + T cells plays an important role in protecting against strains and subtypes of influenza viruses. Like antibodies, influenza virus internal proteins may be detected by cells of CD8 + T. Given that these inner proteins do not experience rapid antigenic transition, CD8 + T cells may provide cross-protection against a wide variety of specific strains of influenza virus. Pre-existing influenza virus-derived CD8 + T cells also received defense against severe disease during the 1957 and 2009 influenza pandemics (Slepushkin, 1959; McMichael et al., 1983; Epstein, 2006; Sridhar et al., 2013; Hayward et al., 2015). Additionally, seasonally mediated influenza-specific CD8 + T cells can cross-react with novel potentially pandemic avian influenza viruses and promote faster recovery in patients following low pathogenic H7N9 avian influenza virus infections. The discovery of retained CD8 + T cell peptides in the 1918 influenza virus 'viral protein sequences and the capacity of the 2009 H1N1 pandemic influenza virus to remember influenza-specific CD8 + T cells, cross-reacting with the 1918 H1N1 influenza virus, suggest that pre-existing CD8 + T cells should be protective against severe infection with the 1918 H1N1 influenza virus specification. Among very young children (age 0–4 years), CD8 + T cells could not have been suitable due to a lack of access to prior influenza viruses (Bodewes et al., 2011a; Sauerbrei et al., 2014). Similarly, in older people (> 65 years), immunosenescence could have impaired the function of CD8 + T cells. This can be clarified by the elevated mortality found during seasonal epidemics (U-shaped curve) in the youngest and oldest age classes.

However, people between the ages of 15 and 65, who endured the largest disease burden during the pandemic of 1918, are considered to exhibit the "gold-standard" immune response, with optimum cross-reactive CD8 + T cell responses. The lack of defensive immunity in this age group is unlikely to be related to the assumption that heterosubtypic immunity is short-lived, as recent reports of the survival of influenza virus-specific CD8 + T cells in healthy individuals. This is likely that the retrieval of pre-existing CD8 + T cell-specific influenza virus responses for the highly virulent 1918 pandemic virus was not quick enough, triggering a sudden outbreak of severe illness and mortality within three days. Alternatively, pandemic H1N1 influenza viruses (1918 and 2009) may have suppressed immunogenic RIPK3-driven dendritic cell death needed to elicit an efficient CD8 + T cell response (Hartmann et al., 2017). Furthermore, ethnically defined genetic differences in HLA molecules are likely to have affected cross-reactive CD8 + T cell responses in individuals diagnosed with the influenza virus (Quiñones-Parra et al., 2014). This (combined with other socio-economic factors) will make a few ethnicities more vulnerable to severe influenza virus infections, such as Alaskan Natives and Indigenous Australians. Nonetheless, in such groups, alarmingly high morbidity and mortality levels were found during the 1918 (Ahmed et al., 2007) and 2009 pandemics (La Ruche et al., 2009; Flint et al., 2010). Likewise, it is interesting to notice that the 1918 virus matrix protein also contained extra-epitopic amino acid residues consistent with the escape of CD8 + T cells from the pre-existing influenza virus (van de Sandt et al., 2015b), a trend not found in the comparatively mild 2009 pandemic influenza virus (van de Sandt et al., 2018a, b).

Finally, it is important to note that the highest rates of influenza virus infection were found in 1918 among school-age children (age 5–15). This increased infection risk; however, it arose when high morbidity was not present (Shanks and Brundage, 2012; Mamelund et al., 2016). Accordingly, school-age children are considered to be in a "honeymoon phase" of superior immunity, exhibiting enhanced tolerance to numerous bacterial and viral pathogens (Ahmed et al., 2007). Given the reality that it contains crucial knowledge for producing successful immune responses to influenza viruses, the processes underlying such a superior immunity remain mostly unexplored.

In this study, we would like to propose an additional hypothesis that could have influenced the effectiveness of the cross-reactive cellular immune response and may have led to the increased mortality of young adults in 1918; namely, immune suppression arising from recent infections with measles (Moss et al., 2004; Griffin, 2010; de Vries et al., 2012; Mina et al., 2015). Measles epidemics were widely recorded in the late 19th and early 20th centuries (Cliff et al., 1983; Duncan et al., 1997; Shulman et al., 2009; Shanks et al., 2011a, 2014), including major measles, the outbreak in US military camps during the winter of 1917–18 (Shanks et al., 2014; Morens and Taubenberger, 2015). During the years before the influenza pandemic of 1918, the elderly population would have undergone measles outbreak during their youth, and their protection should have protected them from contracting measles. However, in the years leading to the influenza pandemic of 1918, infants and young adults may have been immunologically vulnerable to measles without previous measles infections. Recent findings have shown that the measles virus infects recollection T lymphocytes, contributing to apoptosis and sustained immune suppression up to 3 years after initial diagnosis with measles (Moss et al., 2004; Griffin, 2010; de Vries et al., 2012; Mina et al., 2015). Influenza virus-specific CTL responses may also be reduced in young people that had undergone a measles outbreak throughout the years preceding the influenza pandemic of 1918, which could have raised their vulnerability to a severe influenza outbreak. The mixture of immunosuppression regeneration and infection with an unusually extremely virulent virus may have led to severe inflammation associated with pathology through a system best recognized as the Inflammatory Syndrome of Immune Reconstitution (IRIS) (Hirsch et al., 2004; Morens and Fauci, 2007; Shulman et al., 2009; Barber et al., 2012). Whether recent infections with measles ultimately lead to immunosuppression of influenza-specific T-cell responses, resulting in higher vulnerability to serious influenza virus infections and possible IRIS, or contributed to dampening CD8 + T-cell immunopathology remains a significant field of future study. Luckily, measles vaccinations are now readily accessible and have dramatically decreased measles occurrence worldwide (Moss and Griffin, 2012; Perry et al., 2014; Mina et al., 2015). However, a major problem for potential influenza virus pandemics is the elevated amount of measles outbreaks in recent years and the rising vaccination levels.

Together, these results indicate that the age of an individual (and the associated differences in their immune response) played an essential role in deciding the outcome of the disease in the context of pandemic influenza virus infections. In 2009, when identifying priority individuals for the vaccine, age, and preexisting humoral immunity were taken into account. In 2009, the elderly population became less vulnerable to extreme influenza (Dawood et al., 2012), as they were covered by cross-reactive antibodies and CD8 + T cells acquired through previous seasonal infections, including pre-1957 antigenic A / H1N1 virus (Yu et al., 2008; Hancock et al., 2009; Ikonen et al., 2010). Depending on these results, instead of misdirecting to the usual high-risk group: the elderly (National Center for Respiratory Diseases, CDC, and Centers for Disease and Prevention (CDC), 2009), the first small 2009 influenza vaccine supplies were distributed to younger citizens. Improving the cross-reactive reaction of CD8 + T cells to influenza vaccinations and natural infections remains a primary research priority for the future (Clemens et al., 2018). It includes an appreciation of the role of CD8 + T cells in ethnically diverse populations and different age groups (Clemens et al., 2018).

## Genetic Differences

In addition to the function of humoral and cellular immunity, there is growing evidence that suggests that human genetic variations contribute to differences in the severity of influenza virus infections. For example, several single-nucleotide polymorphisms (SNPs) were closely linked to extreme pneumonia during the influenza pandemic of 2009. This contained SNPs in the interferon reaction factor 7 genes (Ciancanelli et al., 2015), Fc fragment of immunoglobulin G, low-affinity IIA, receptor (Zúñiga et al., 2012), RPA interacting protein (Zúñiga et al., 2012), complement component 1q subcomponent binding protein (Zúñiga et al.,

2012), CD55 (Zhou et al., 2012), IL-1α (Liu et al., 2013), IL-1β (Liu et al., 2013), surfactant protein B g g Unfortunately, insufficient evidence is accessible to determine that either of the above SNPs affected the mortality differences in 1918. Defining increasing SNPs impart enhanced vulnerability to serious influenza remains an important feature of pandemic preparedness for influenza, as it can help warn increasing communities that they are most at risk for serious disease.

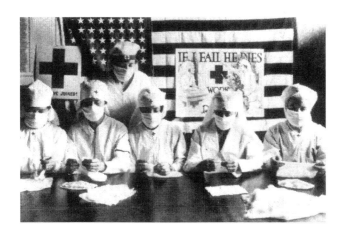

## Malnutrition

Host nutritional status has long been recognized as an important factor in multiple infectious disease outcomes (Cohen, 2000). Throughout India in 1918, the effects of starvation and drought were especially evident in the magnitude of influenza. The influenza pandemic of 1918 hit India amid a widespread drought, reducing the productivity of several essential food crops (Mills, 1986). Consequently, during 1918, many North-Western, Western, and Central Indian provinces endured famine (Mills, 1986). It was these areas that experienced the highest death rates for influenza in 1918 (Mills, 1986). Although of the pandemic's unprecedented age range, those who fell to the epidemic were usually young adults who made up the bulk of the agricultural workforce (Mills, 1986). The ensuing labor crisis helped only to intensify the severity of the influenza pandemic (Mills, 1986). The specific processes by which poverty and famine increase influenza intensity remain to be established.

Experimental findings, however, indicate that starvation not only suppresses the host's immune response to the influenza virus but may also promote the development of new viral strains, which display enhanced pathogenicity compared to the initial parental strain (Beck et al., 2004).

Undernutrition (often exacerbated by ongoing civil war) remains a problem for the twenty-first century and beyond influenza pandemics. It was believed that severe malnutrition led to the high morbidity and mortality seen in Guatemalan children during the influenza pandemic of 2009 (Reyes et al., 2010). Climate change may contribute to crop failures that would exacerbate any future food shortages. However, we will face a "double risk" of starvation in every potential influenza virus pandemic, whereby a proportion of the world's population will experience severe disease due to undernutrition, and a portion of the world's population will experience severe illness due to overnutrition. In particular, it is now well accepted that obesity raises one's likelihood of getting diagnosed with an influenza virus infection and dying from it (Morgan et al., 2010; Louie et al., 2011; Van Kerkhove et al., 2011). The possibility that obesity prevents all virus-specific responses to CD8 + T cells and antibody responses to the seasonal influenza vaccine is maybe even more troubling (Sheridan et al., 2012). Therefore, the threat of potential influenza pandemics is not just to protect those afflicted by undernutrition (particularly in light of the growing climate change problem) but also the number of people living with obesity.

## Underlying Infections

### Co-infection with bacterial pathogens

Historical autopsy findings and analysis of the lung tissue parts from 1918 to 19 influenza case data revealed that the cause of death was not predominant viral pneumonia for a large number of cases (Brundage and Shanks, 2008; Morens et al., 2008; Chien et al., 2009), Rather, such people are led to a secondary bacterial infection, which is often triggered by bacteria such as Streptococcus pneumonia, Haemophilus influenza, Staphylococcus aureus, and Streptococcus pyogenes (Morens et al., 2008). H. Influenzae was found so often in influenza patients that it was sometimes identified as the source of the pandemic (and was thus named as that) (Hildreth, 1991). Throughout the 1918 epidemic, the role of secondary bacterial infections is consistent with epidemiological findings that although influenza virus attack levels were comparable among soldiers and civilians in 1918, mortality rates among freshly arriving soldiers were far higher (Shanks et al., 2016b). The unhygienic conditions in the army camps led to recurrent bacterial infections, especially among new army recruits who were immunologically naive.

Therefore, recent army recruits were more prone to acquire a deadly secondary bacterial pneumonia after an influenza virus infection than people or long-serving veterans (Shanks et al., 2010, 2016b). Numerous animal laboratory experiments have repeated these findings, demonstrating that co-infection with the influenza virus and bacterial pathogens results in the high intensity of illness relative to any pathogen infection (Brightman, 1935; Glover, 1941; Francis and de Torregrosa, 1945; Harford et al., 1946; Wilson et al., 1947; Short et al., 2012a, 2013). Various pathways have been suggested to clarify this synergism between virus and bacteria (McCullers, 2006; McAuley et al., 2007; Smith et al., 2013; Hrincius et al., 2015). Such involve, but are not limited to, decreased mucociliary clearance of inhaled bacteria following influenza virus infection, bacterial adhesion to the basement membrane (Morens et al., 2008; Taubenberger et al., 2012; Chertow and Memoli, 2013) and influenza virus-exposed sialic acids (McCullers and Bartmess, 2003; Peltola et al., 2005), viral changes to the immune response of the host (Navarin, 2003) Most importantly, laboratory findings show that influenza viruses not only increase the frequency of secondary bacterial infections but also improve S propagation. Diavatopoulos et al. (2010; Short et al., 2012b).

In addition to co-infections with bacterial pathogens, such as S. Chronic bacterial pneumonia diseases, such as Mycobacterium tuberculosis leading to influenza mortality differences during the 1918 pandemic. For example, evidence from a Swiss sanatorium during the 1918 epidemic showed that the probability of death from influenza among patients with tuberculosis (TB) was higher than that of non-TB (Oei and Nishiura, 2012). Likewise, people with TB were 2.2 times more likely than non-TB individuals residing in the same household to develop the influenza virus of 1918 (Noymer and Garenne, 2000; Noymer, 2011). A synergistic M-relationship Experimental experiment has also provided

211

help to tuberculosis and influenza viruses (Redford et al., 2014). In 1918, the incidence of TB in young adults may have led to the dramatic "W-shaped" death curve correlated with the influenza pandemic of 1918 (Oei and Nishiura 2012).

Due to bacterial co-infections, severe complications and morbidity were not exclusive to the influenza pandemic of 1918. Instead, in the influenza pandemics of 1957, 1968 and 2009, bacterial co-infections were also reported, but to a smaller degree than in 1918 (Oswald et al., 1958; Robertson et al., 1958; Louria et al., 1959; Oseasohn et al., 1959; Chertow and Memoli, 2013; Joseph et al., 2013). TB was also reported as a contributing factor in the occurrence of serious illness during the 2009 influenza pandemic (Morales et al., 2017). Fortunately, unlike in 1918, the extent of bacterial infections during the recent influenza pandemics was possibly reduced by antibiotic usage, modern medical care, and the availability of bacterial vaccines [such as pneumococcal polysaccharide and H. Oswald et al., 1958; Robertson et al., 1958; Louria et al., 1959; Madhi et al., 2004; Wahl et al., 2018). However, as antibiotic resistance levels begin to increase and as pathogens such as methicillin-resistant S start to grow, Aureus (MRSA) and multidrug tolerant M. (Memoli et al., 2008). Tuberculosis (Zumla et al., 2013; Millard et al., 2015) is becoming more widespread, so we may, in the future, face situations in which antibiotics become unsuccessful in treating bacterial infections. This would have clear the severe implications for every potential pandemic influenza virus (Memoli et al., 2008). Not only reducing antibiotic tolerance but also engaging in the development of novel drugs and safe therapeutic methods for bacterial infections must be considered an urgent priority.

## Malaria

In addition to Individuals with bacterial co-infections, the mortality of malaria-infected people during the 1918

213

influenza pandemic was significantly higher (Langford and Storey, 1992; Afkhami, 2003; Shanks, 2015). While the underlying mechanism is not well known, a procoagulant state caused by malaria could play a role in increasing inflammation and resulting in clinical outcomes (Shanks, 2015).

Chemopreventive strategies have today lowered the burden of disease associated with malaria, and new strategies for eradication are being created. Malaria, though, also induces significant international morbidity and mortality, there is ever-increasing medication resistance, and modern malaria vaccines are yet to have long-lasting population-level benefits (Ashlcy ct al., 2018). Before the creation and introduction of successful control measures, malaria resistant areas remain at high risk for high mortality throughout the influenza pandemic.

## Non-pharmaceutical interventions

In 1918, numerous methods were implemented to restrict influenza virus transmission and cure sick patients. While all of these approaches were of little to no use, they provide valuable lessons for twenty-first-century influenza pandemic preparedness.

## Maritime Quarantine

Many countries placed stringent quarantine controls on all new ships in 1918 as the second outbreak of influenza became evident (Johnson, 2006). Those efforts were mostly ineffective (Johnson, 2006). Quarantine measures were either enforced too late, and the virus was already prevalent in the country or quarantine was violated by non-symptomatic infectious individuals (Crosby, 1976; Tomkins, 1992). Thus, countries such as the U.K. And South Africa opposed maritime quarantine as ineffective and impractical (Blakely, 2006; Johnson, 2006). However, Australia placed the marine quarantine before reports were made of any victims of the second wave. Both incoming vessels had to be inspected before disembarking by Commonwealth Quarantine authorities. This quarantine shielded Australia from the pandemic's second wave until December 1918 when the quarantine was eventually broken. Maritime quarantine thus helped protect Australia from the worst of the pandemic (Crosby, 2003; Johnson, 2006) and indirectly helped protect some Pacific Islands, which relied on Australian supply ships (Shanks et al., 2018).

The most striking example of this was the disparity in mortality between US Samoa and Western Samoa. The US Samoa governor has placed a stringent maritime quarantine in American Samoa in 1918 (Shanks, and Brundage, 2013). This quarantine prohibited influenza from reaching the country, and in America Samoa, no deaths of influenza were reported in the 1918 pandemic (Johnson, 2006; Shanks and Brundage,

2013). This was compared actively with the neighboring western Samoa (located ~100 km away), which did not observe strict maritime quarantine (Tomkins, 1992; Shanks and Brundage, 2013). As a result, the New Zealand delivery ship, the Talune, poisoned Western Samoa, and it is reported that more than one-fifth of the populace died of influenza (Tomkins, 1992).

In the last century, global transport has experienced a significant transformation, with ships being substituted by the quicker and more commonly used air transportation. The increase of commercial air traffic helps understand the accelerated global outbreak of the more recent 1957, 1968, and 2009 influenza pandemic in the absence of large military troop movements (Rvachev and Longini, 1985; Hufnagel et al., 2004; Khan et al., 2009; Bajardi et al., 2011; Lemey et al., 2014). However, it is impossible in maritime isolation to play a part in curbing the outbreak of any potential influenza pandemic. In 2009, though, officials sought to restrict influenza transmission by utilizing the modern-day version of maritime quarantine: airport entry screening, Sadly, in 2009, a study of arriving passengers at Sydney airport revealed that airport screening only had a sensitivity of 6.67 percent in identifying influenza-infected patients, thus costing ~50,000AUD per testing (Gunaratnam et al., 2014). This limited effectiveness and undoubtedly illustrates the reality that people afflicted with influenza virus may become infectious before becoming symptomatic (Hollingsworth et al., 2006). Therefore, it is doubtful that airport entry screening can control the transmission of influenza through international air traffic. Alternatively, progressing models (e.g., determining which transportation paths are more susceptible to disease spread) and various outreach strategies (e.g., increasing public consciousness of the dangers of traveling with an infected individual) is likely to play a more significant role in future pandemic preparedness.

## Mass Gatherings

In addition to limiting maritime travel, many cities introduced necessary non-pharmaceutical measures in 1918 to prevent the transmission of viruses. This included the introduction of limits on social occasions where communication could occur from individual to individual. As a result, colleges, theatres, temples, and dance halls were closed, while public events such as marriages and funerals were prohibited to avoid overcrowding (Frost, 1919; Johnson, 2006; Bootsma and Ferguson, 2007; Hatchett et al., 2007). In communities that quickly introduced such non-pharmaceutical measures within a few days of reporting the first local deaths, the peak mortality risk was lower compared to those who waited a few weeks to respond (Bootsma and Ferguson, 2007; Hatchett et al., 2007). The pace of removing such measures also impacted infant mortality (Bootsma and Ferguson, 2007; Hatchett et al., 2007). Therefore, limitations on people's meetings helped to limit the spread of influenza virus, as soon as those limitations were eased (typically within 2-8 weeks of implementation), effective viral spread started again (Hatchett et al., 2007).

Following the outbreak of Mexico's 2009 pandemic influenza virus, a compulsory school closure for 18 days was implemented in the crowded Mexico City area (Chowell et al., 2011). This was combined with an influenza transmission decrease of 29–37 percent (Chowell et al., 2011). Similarly, a 25 percent reduction in influenza virus spread occurred in Hong Kong after the closing of secondary schools from June 11 to July 10, 2009 (Wu et al., 2010). Just like in 1918, however, the length of such intervention strategies impacted their efficacy, and in the autumn of 2009, there was a significant rise in influenza incidence in 32 Mexican states, a span that coincided with schools opening for the autumn term (Chowell et al., 2011).

## Facemasks and Hygiene

Facemasks were a popular preventive measure used during the Pandemic of 1918. While people were unsure of the pandemic's etiologic agent, the assumption was that it was an infectious illness that should be avoided by wearing a facemask (Crosby, 1976). Accordingly, several towns and areas, including Guatemala City, San Francisco, and some Japanese prefectures, made it mandatory to wear a facemask in public locations, and various task forces and awareness programs were set up to implement this legislation (Crosby, 1976; Rice and Palmer, 1993; Rice, 2011). However, to be moderately successful against the influenza virus, a facemask must be (i) use at all times, (ii) correctly designed and installed, and (iii) made of suitable content. Such criteria were often not fulfilled by the medical gauze masks of 1918 (Crosby, 1976). Thus, Ontario, Canada's mortality rate (where it was optional to wear a mask) was not significantly different from Alberta, Canada (where mask-wearing was imposed by law) (MacDougall 2007). Influenza deaths in Alberta began to grow well after mask-wearing had been legalized by law, suggesting that wearing a facemask in 1918 was not enough to avoid influenza deaths (World Health Organization Writing Group et al., 2006).

Proper hygiene (e.g., frequent hand washing) would also have helped to limit the influenza virus spread during the 1918 pandemic since influenza viruses are mouth-to-face transmissible (World Health Organization Writing Group et al., 2006; Thomas et al., 2014). Thus, the traditional Japanese attitude to illness and disease may have led to a lower national pandemic mortality in 1918–19, as Japanese children are told to remove their shoes and wash their hands immediately they arrive home (Rice and Palmer, 1993).

Facemasks and handwashing/hand sanitizers were seen as preventive, non-pharmaceutical measures in the context of the modern influenza pandemics. Nevertheless, the use of facemasks was primarily not mandatory during the influenza pandemic of 2009 (CDC, 2009). Instead, the CDC only proposed facemasks for people at higher risk of severe influenza disease or people that were the immediate neighbor of the pandemic virus affected persons (CDC, 2009). Also, the efficacy of facemasks in avoiding influenza virus spread remains uncertain (Cowling et al., 2010), and, as was found in 1918, poor public enforcement dramatically reduces the utility of facemasks in a contemporary pandemic environment (Cowling et al., 2010). These procedures can be of paramount significance to emergency staff who work on the front line of a pandemic and are at high risk of infection. By contrast, hand washing and the use of hand sanitizers (whether or not in combination with wearing a facemask) during the 2009 influenza pandemic had a strong preventive effect (Larson et al., 2012; Suess et al., 2012; Wong et al., 2014).

Such evidence indicates that in any future influenza pandemic, non-pharmaceutical interventions such as social distancing, handwashing/hand sanitizers, and facemasks can buy valuable time before vaccines become widely available. The effectiveness of such measures may, however, rely on their early and continuing implementation, and also on the ability of people to comply. The 1918 pandemic has demonstrated that while voluntary interventions are more successful as citizens have a poor appetite for compulsory safety initiatives (Spinney, 2017). However, a behavioral analysis found that while people were offered autonomy-supportive guidance relative to guided orders, they were more inclined to wear a facemask (Chan et al., 2015).

## Medical interventions, therapies and vaccines: then and now

The influenza pandemic of 1918 arose at a time in history when control of infectious diseases had become a scientific profession's practical priority (Tomkins, 1992; Johnson, 2006). Initiatives in public safety have also proved effective in reducing disease transmissions, such as cholera and TB (Hildreth, 1991; Tomkins, 1992; Tognotti, 2003). Initially, there was nothing to say that an influenza epidemic could not be managed successfully (Hildreth, 1991; Tomkins, 1992; Tognotti, 2003). Nevertheless, the etiological agent of the influenza pandemic of 1918 remained a mystery given the drastic developments in microbiology in recent decades. Several specific clinical and prevention measures are tried in the absence of clear knowledge regarding the pandemic's causative factor. People also dealt with medicines (including Asprin) and home-made treatments such as mustard poultice, quinine, nicotine, beef tea, zinc sulfate inhalation, morphine, saltwater, and alcohol (Rice and Palmer, 1993; Johnson, 2006; Starko, 2009; Keeling, 2010). Traditional Eastern medicine, such as Japanese Kanpo medication (consisting of herbal medicines supplemented by green tea) may have had a positive impact by inducing abruptness (helping to reduce fever), raising rates of vitamin C and restoring missing fluids (Palmer and Rice, 1992; Rice and Palmer, 1993). Furthermore, the usage of Traditional Chinese Medicine in some people could have minimized the frequency of influenza infections (Kobayashi et al., 1999; Cheng and Leung, 2007; Chen et al., 2011). However, in terms of successful medical and prophylactic procedures, nothing became available for the most part. Also, nursing care has shown to have helped in patient rehabilitation, especially those suffering from secondary bacterial pneumonia (Robinson, 1990; Rice and Palmer, 1993). In comparison, death rates in areas lacking health services, such as minefields, were considerably higher (Phimister 1973; Rice and Palmer 1993). Unfortunately, all of those who usually performed these duties either worked abroad or became ill themselves during the 1918–19 pandemic (Crosby, 2003; Keeling, 2010; Shanks et al., 2011b).

Today the detection of the influenza etiologic agent has significantly increased the pace and precision of diagnosis. Quick and extremely effective molecular diagnostic methods have increasingly substituted the labor-intensive and time-consuming "gold standard" system of cell culture for diagnosing influenza virus infections (Ellis and Zambon, 2002), which enables quick isolation of infected persons. The risk of identification of possible pandemic viruses has been significantly enhanced by examining the human and animal virus and isolates viral genomes for the presence of mutations that improve human adaptation or virulence.

However, in the event of an influenza virus pandemic, we should introduce all anti-viral medications and vaccinations. Antivirals (such as oseltamivir and zanamivir neuraminidase inhibitors) can be employed as a treatment in critically sick patients, but can also be used prophylactically in epidemic cases (Cooper et al., 2003; Hayden et al., 2004; De Clercq, 2006; Zambon, 2014; Krammer et al., 2018). At present, both oseltamivir and zanamivir are vulnerable to possibly pandemic influenza viruses (such as avian H7N9 and H5N1 viruses) (Herfst et al., 2012). Nonetheless, some H5N1 isolates have found gained tolerance to oseltamivir (De Clercq, 2006). Likewise, tolerance to oseltamivir is reported to grow in H7N9 viruses within two days of treatment (Hay and Hayden, 2013). Such results indicate that antivirals will be utilized judiciously in the case of any potential influenza virus pandemic, and the existence of drug-resistant viral forms should be closely watched.

Vaccines for the influenza virus also played an important role in reducing the morbidity and mortality associated with seasonal influenza. Unfortunately, for an antigenic distinct influenza virus with a novel subtype such as A / H5N1 or A / H7N9, antibodies released by seasonal influenza vaccinations do not offer safety (De Jong et al., 2000). In fact, existing seasonal inactivated influenza vaccinations will also inhibit the activation of cross-reactive CD8 + T cell responses, which are our main defense in the case of a pandemic and may thus prove to be a double-edged sword (Bodewes et al., 2009a, b, 2011b, c). The rapid development of vaccines remains a threat to potential pandemic influenza viruses (World Health Organisation, 2005; Rockman and Gray, 2010; Pada and Tambyah, 2011). This became especially clear during the 2009 pandemic, as adequate doses of the virus vaccine became accessible only in October 2009, well and truly after the epidemic had exploded worldwide (Butler, 2010). The development of vaccines in a pandemic scenario

229

could be more complicated by the possibility that some avian influenza viruses may destroy the embryonic chicken eggs required to manufacture the vaccine (Tumpey et al., 2005). In tandem with alternate manufacturing models for vaccines, innovative vaccine approaches are necessary to increase the development of vaccines and prevent these issues (Schotsaert and García-Sastre, 2014). But the gold standard for pandemic preparedness remains an influenza vaccine that delivers long-lasting, wide-spectrum protection. Previously analyzed how fundamental humoral and cellular biology and human clinical evidence should be interpreted for the introduction of a standardized influenza vaccine (Clemens et al., 2018).

## Prevention Against Further Pandemic Outbreak

If in future, we had a global influenza pandemic akin to the size and virulence of the one that struck a century ago — in 1918, about 50 million people were affected by the Spanish flu — it would cost our modern economy an estimated $3 billion. And, the study states, "If today a comparable contagion happened with a population four times larger and also traveled less time than 36 hours anywhere in the world, 50-80 million people could perish." To avert such an outcome, the report offers numerous recommendations — some scientific, some financial, some social. Below are five standout suggestions:

- Heads of government can spend large amounts of money in preparedness as an integral part of national and global security in any country.

- All countries should develop a system to share genome sequences of all new pathogens without hesitation.

- Public health systems will create trust in residents so that in the case of an epidemic, they would be more willing to obey guidelines.

- Health officials should include women in preparation and decision-making, mainly because the plurality of clinicians are women, and their participation promotes the adoption of policies and strategies.

- Donors will boost support for the poorest countries and address financing gaps for their national health-security action plans.

## Concluding Remarks

It is estimated that if today a pandemic influenza virus of the same virulence and attack intensity as the influenza virus of 1918 were to reappear, mortality could increase to 21–147 million (Murray et al., 2006; Madhav, 2013). Nevertheless, the elevated morbidity and mortality levels correlated with the influenza pandemic of 1918 arose from a dynamic interplay of variables that are inherent to the infection itself, the immune response of the host, and the social context in which the pandemic occurred. So, this same mix of variables is impossible to replicate in the future. But, a comprehensive understanding of the factors contributing to the magnitude of the pandemic of 1918 plays a vital role in our readiness for the next influenza pandemic.

# CHAPTER SIX

# POSSIBILITY OF FUTURE PANDEMIC

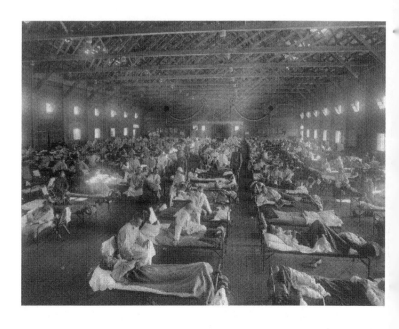

As humans regularly cross borders and live closer together, the risk of an outbreak is greater than ever. Experts claim that climate change and civil strife add to the danger too. It might take only one cough, one hug, one-touch, or even one bite to

change not only your life but everyone's life around you —
and for months or even years.

The closer these people are to you in most cases, the higher
the risk. But that's not always so easy. The underlying risk: an
infectious epidemic. Experts in public health agree that we
are at higher risk than ever before of witnessing large-scale
outbreaks and global pandemics such as those we've
experienced before: Spanish Flu 1918, SARS, swine flu,
Ebola and Zika

During the 2014-16 Ebola epidemic, more than 28,000 people
were infected and more than 11,000 deaths. And as of 10
March, 84 countries reported transmission of Zika. The
disease was identified in the 1940s but had its first outbreak
in Micronesia in 2007, and more recently began spreading
toward the end of 2015.

The emergence of the virus is unexpected at any time, and the size is unprecedented, making the planet vulnerable.

Experts are unanimous in the conviction that most definitely, the next outbreak contender will arrive as a shock — so we need to be ready.

"We're only as safe in the world as the weakest country," said Jimmy Whitworth, an international public health instructor at the London School of Hygiene & Tropical Medicine. In a vulnerable state with so many health systems and economies, that means we are far from free.

"Infectious diseases do not honor frontiers," he added. Every month, he said, the World Health Organization is alerted to hundreds of minor outbreaks which it is monitoring and utilizing to forecast the likelihood of a bigger issue.

"There is all the time, all over the world, little clusters of outbreaks occurring," Whitworth said.

But even with infections disregarding borders and forming their lines of the battle against humanity, he claims the way we live now is what exposes us to risk.

"Many aspects of modern life put us at higher risk. We're more equipped than ever," he points out, referencing the Global Disease Warning and Response Network International Health Laws and countries with regional rapid response teams — such as the United States, the United Kingdom, and China — able to cope with any disaster.

## SEVEN (7) REASONS FUTURE PANDEMIC MAY OCCUR

### 1. Growing populations and urbanization

The facts about urban life are simple: you live, eat, work, and move closer to people than in any rural area, thus providing greater opportunities for the spread of disease by air, mosquitoes, or unclean water. As populations intensify, so do the number of urban dwellers, with the United Nations predicting that by 2050 66 percent of the world's people will be residing in urban areas.

More residents in cities can "put a strain on sanitation," said David Heymann, director of the Chatham House think tank at the Centre for Global Health Security beyond the proximity of humans, "this is the second cause of infection," he said, and a third is increasing demand for food, forcing farmers to produce more grain, and more animals, allowing them to live near those animals as well.

Cattle are vectors for other illnesses, including tuberculosis bovine cattle and African sleeping sickness (trypanosomiasis), and avian flu poultry. With citizens shifting from — and from — rural environments to urban ones more frequently, their likelihood of being sick and instead of living in near quarters with others also enhances the risk for transmitting stuff.

## 2. Encroaching into new environments

As the number of inhabitants grows, so will the amount of land available for them to be housed. Populations are spreading to regions historically uninhabited, such as wetlands. With new areas, new species, and eventually, new diseases coming in contact.

For example, "Lassa fever is happening because people are living in the forest and killing it for farming," Heymann said.

Lassa fever is a viral disease that spreads through contact with infected rodent feces. It may induce fever and hemorrhage in different sections of the body, including the nose and lips. Transmission from individual to individual is also feasible, but less regular. Outbreaks typically occur in West Africa, with the occurrences in Nigeria after 2016 higher than anticipated.

Heymann states that Lassa is one example of people residing around woodland areas where contaminated rodents live. Still, degradation of such habitats for farming leaves the animals nowhere to go — other than living with humans. "It's not feasible for the rats that stay there to get food and move into human arcas for food," he added.

## 3. Climate change

The research appears to demonstrate that climate change is contributing to further hot storms and flooding incidents, providing further possibilities for waterborne diseases like cholera and disease vectors like mosquitoes in new areas.

"Flooding happens with greater frequency," Heymann said, in which the probability of outbreaks is raised.

According to the World Health Organisation, climate change is expected to cause around 250,000 extra deaths each year from heat stress, starvation, and the spread of infectious diseases such as malaria between 2030 and 2050.

The possibility of an epidemic is strong with disease carriers such as mosquitoes increasingly able to survive in new unregulated areas.

Whitworth cited Angola's latest yellow fever epidemic, which has killed over 350 individuals. He clarified that any yellow fever virus might have been spread by mosquitoes in China as

China's staff returned home from Angola. Although, the absence of staff in winter indicated that the insects weren't around to spread by bites.

The increasing population of the globe provides greater potential for the disease to spread by soil, mosquitoes, or unclean water, particularly in urban areas. The UN estimates that by 2050, 66 percent of the world's people will be residing in metropolitan areas.

## 4. Global Voyage

"We are prone to accelerated sailing," Whitworth said. Foreign visitor arrivals in 2015 hit an unprecedented nearly 1.2 billion, 50 million more than in 2014, according to the United Nations World Tourism Organisation. This was the sixth year in a row of above-average production. And with more people going at all stages, there are more ways to catch a lift for pathogens.

"Infectious agents severally fly inside their incubation span in humans," Heymann said. An incubation period is an interval between the emergence of signs and the infection, indicating that people may spread the disease even if they do not seem to be ill.

The 2003 SARS (severe acute respiratory syndrome) pandemic is believed to have begun with Dr. Liu Jianlun, who on a trip to Huang Xingchu in China acquired signs of the airborne virus, and later returned to see relatives in Hong Kong. He polluted his hotel and relatives. He was then admitted to the hospital and died, as did one of his friends.

Around 4,000 cases and 550 deaths from SARS could be linked back to Liu's stay in Hong Kong within less than four months. More than 8,000 other citizens in more than 30 countries worldwide were sick.

Yet Heymann emphasizes that "those who transmit illness by travel are not just humans." Infections occur by plants, fruit, and livestock shipped through nations. "This is also commerce," he said, referring to malaria at the airport, where people at airports were contaminated with malaria by mosquitoes that hitched a ride on a plane or in fruit.

He also identified bird flu that was halted in 2004 on the Belgian border in Thai eagles exchanged as pets. Guinea rats imported through the United States as livestock throughout 2003 harbored monkeypox diseases, he said, and then infected prairie dogs, and ultimately humans.

**5. Legal conflict**

"When a health-care network is unwilling to manage an epidemic, there is chaos," he added. He assumes that bad hygiene is no acceptable argument everywhere, including in evolving environments, because it is easy to sterilize and hand-wash.

But if a nation is on the verge of civil war, the failure to cope with an extreme and unexpected issue like an epidemic might bring the population on their knees — and enable the infection to thrive.

"Nations may be fully devastated by diseases," Whitworth stated, referencing the 2014 Ebola crisis in which Sierra Leone, Guinea, and Liberia were "near to collapse." Political instability had ravaged all three nations, leaving their economic and health systems in desperate need of repair – yet unprepared for a big infection.

This issue, coupled with human migration between these three countries and many more internationally indicated that Ebola could spread even though thousands of outbreaks in previous years were self-contained in the neighboring

Democratic Republic of Congo and mostly resolved themselves. "If (an infection) stays local, then it will flame out," Heymann said. "The public is studying what to do."

## 6. Fewer doctors and nurses in outbreak regions

In addition to weak health systems, nations with a higher risk of diseases — namely, more developing settings — often have fewer doctors and nurses to treat the population. Many have moved elsewhere to search for better prospects.

"We have to treat this as a fact," Heymann said, adding that some countries are now promoting young medical talent to move to new places.

"It's hard to handle the relocation of health care workers," he added. Yet initiatives and approaches are ongoing to address this by "task-shifting," moving responsibilities to new groups and preparing them to deliver care, such as community health workers. "Communities need to be adaptive," he said, so assigning tasks to individuals at all levels, as a new epidemic strikes, could make a good team available.

## 7. Faster information

In the information age, new levels of contact bring yet increased levels of fear and various means of spreading it, experts believe.

While the majority of small outbreaks might once have been relatively unnoticed to communities farther out from the epicenter, today's people are more educated than ever. They need fast-flowing, transparent, reliable information.

Google has been using symptom searches to determine better where an outbreak, such as flu, may occur.

"The world is looking for an authority," Heymann said, who assumes that position is held by the WHO but needs to be faster and more open with the information. The organization has been criticized for being too slow to respond to the 2014 Ebola epidemic and not preparing for it."But social networking has become active ... so it's an area that is difficult-to-control," he said.

Multiple people's posting and influencing of information will affect advertising, and what people read and think, Heymann added. Not everyone might be evil, he said, but the argument is that it may affect the way information travels, potentially stirring up fear and stigma.

"Not every internet or social media information is reliable," said Mark Feinberg, chairman of the Scientific Advisory Committee of the newly formed Coalition for Epidemic Preparedness Innovations. "It's critically necessary to provide accurate information to the public." Launched in January, the initiative must discuss the surprise nature of diseases and epidemics and try to prevent them, rather than respond to them.

Made in the USA
Middletown, DE
20 May 2020

95490153R00149